Alopecia Areata

Alopecia Areata

Understanding and Coping with Hair Loss

Wendy Thompson, M.A.

Jerry Shapiro, M.D.

Foreword by Vera H. Price, M.D.

THE JOHNS HOPKINS UNIVERSITY PRESS
BALTIMORE AND LONDON

©1996 The Johns Hopkins University Press
All rights reserved. Published 1996
Printed in the United States of America on acid-free recycled paper
05 04 03 02 01 99 98 97 96   5 4 3 2 1

The Johns Hopkins University Press
2715 North Charles Street
Baltimore, Maryland 21218-4319
The Johns Hopkins Press Ltd., London

Library of Congress Cataloging-in-Publication Data will be found at
the end of this book.

A catalog record for this book is available from the British Library.

ISBN 0-8018-5352-4
ISBN 0-8018-6472-0 (pbk)

This book is dedicated to everyone with Alopecia Areata

Your vulnerability turned to strength
Your despair turned to hope
Your fear turned to courage
Your knowledge turned to self-esteem

W.T.

Contents

Foreword

Alopecia areata is a challenging disease. The sudden appearance of patches of hair loss on the scalp, or the loss of all hair on the scalp and elsewhere, can be an overwhelming experience. Alopecia areata alters the lives of those who have it, as well as the lives of family and friends. The alteration in one's life can ultimately be a positive one. Some people accept their condition with remarkable composure and inner strength, and inspire all those around them with their vitality, sensitivity, and humor. More commonly, however, the road to regaining self-confidence is a long one—though very worthwhile. The experience of living with this disease, and coping with its emotional pain, often produces the most successful, productive, and generous human beings. For this reason, it is important to help every child, teen, and adult with alopecia areata to stay in the mainstream of life and not postpone doing things "until my hair grows back."

Alopecia areata is capricious. One never knows how long an episode will last—weeks, months, years—before the hair regrows, or when another episode will occur, if ever. Because of this unpredictability, and because those affected are usually otherwise healthy, the first essential step in coping with alopecia areata is to know everything about it. Why me? What caused it? Am I the only one who has this? Does anyone else feel as self-conscious, embarrassed, and depressed as I do? And how can I grow my hair back?

In *Alopecia Areata: Understanding and Coping with Hair Loss,* Wendy Thompson and Dr. Jerry Shapiro provide answers to all these questions. The book is an excellent source of information about the disease and the roller coaster emotional ride that usually accompanies it. Both authors have had a long experience with alopecia areata: Wendy Thompson has it herself, and Dr. Jerry Shapiro has devoted his medical career to treating patients with it and studying new treatments for it. It is the personal perspective that makes this book special and all the more persuasive. The goal is to help people cope and regain control of their lives. And there are practical, helpful suggestions throughout. One of the few predictable aspects of alopecia areata is its unpredictability. This feature is well brought out in the medical chapter, which describes in detail the various ways the condition may present itself, how long it will last, and how it responds to our current treatments. And there is hope for the future with the worldwide research to find the cause and cure.

This book is a pleasure to read because of its intimate style and humor. It will go a long way to help those with alopecia areata.

VERA H. PRICE, M.D.
Professor of Clinical Dermatology,
University of California, San Francisco, and
Chairman of the Medical Advisory Board,
National Alopecia Areata Foundation

Preface

Dr. Shapiro and I wrote this book to help people with alopecia areata cope with their condition by explaining what hair loss is and how it affects people. Coping in a world that discriminates against baldness is not simple, and neither is the message of this book. What fills these pages is the latest medical information and treatments, strategies for coping, and other tools to help. The ultimate goal of this book is to enhance life.

Over the last forty years, I have had little hair, lots of hair, and no hair. I have worn a wig, gone without a wig, and tried almost every treatment. As I write these words, my hair is growing. I still can't "bat an eyelash" or "raise an eyebrow," but I will one day. So I can laugh and joke. But I know very well that it's no joke to lose your hair. I also know that getting to the point of being able to laugh is a journey worth taking.

Hair carries with it an importance that is only fully understood when you lose it. Still, different people react to hair loss differently. Some get a wig and learn to accept it, some get a wig and never accept it, some find a wig too much bother. For some people, wigs are cover-ups that don't cover up the real issues.

When a person has alopecia areata and the joy in life becomes dependent on the state of his or her hair, that person can end up in emotional turmoil. If self-esteem, self-identity, and even the ability to function are dependent on the condition of our hair, and then something happens to it that is beyond our control, we have to make an adjustment in our thinking. By looking deeply, we will learn that we are not our hair. With hard work, we can make that adjustment in our thinking.

Big issues! This book is written to address these issues. In addition to being a comprehensive guide to the diagnosis and treatment of alopecia areata, it offers coping strategies. More important, it offers to help you live fully the life you choose, regardless of whether you have hair or not.

I was seven years old when I noticed a large bald patch behind my left ear and heard the term *alopecia areata* for the first time. No one else in my world had ever heard it before, either. By the time I was eight, all my hair had fallen out and my world had changed completely. I was bald from head to toe.

What sticks out in my memory is facing the first day of school that fall. I walked out the front door with a very skimpy scarf that didn't cover my head, got half-way down our sidewalk, and turned back. My mother waved her arm slowly and firmly as if to plant some of her inner strength in me, and she said in a kind voice, "You have to go now." I think it was as hard for her as it was for me. In those days, more than forty years ago, this disease was never discussed. By anyone. Ever.

Recently I counted up the days I was teased about my hair as a child—the total was 2,550. Every time I was outside my home, I was teased and stared at until I covered up the problem with a wig and created a new identity. What happened every time I was teased? I felt hurt, helpless, and angry. I ate the words and they ate me. I mastered the skillful art of stuffing down my feelings so I wouldn't feel the pain. Thousands of children have experienced pain like this. The old children's verse that goes "Sticks and stones may break my bones, but names will never hurt me" just isn't true. Names *do* hurt.

By the age of nineteen I was in college, taking courses to become a teacher. Of all my experiences with this disease, of all the years of teasing, the worst incident occurred in a physical education course in college—and it may have been the worst simply because it was the most unjust. What started it was that I asked to be exempted from two sections of the course. Because I was bald and wore a wig I couldn't do the tumbling (although I could have demonstrated the skills privately), and I was unable to "head the ball" for the soccer test.

Heading the ball means bouncing the ball off your forehead, an easy skill to learn without a wig but almost impossible to do while keeping a wig on. (Double-sided tape didn't exist at the time.) I suggested to the instructor that I do a written assignment instead, but the instructor refused to honor my request. So, I took a soccer ball home and for a week I practiced "heading" the ball off my forehead with my wig on. If I hit the ball in exactly the right spot and did not jerk my head, I could do it.

When the day of the test came, I "headed the ball" masterfully in front of the whole class. Outside, I felt a sort of victory, but inside my anger at the injustice left me with deep resentment that I am only now coming to terms with. I lined up my first teaching position before I graduated that spring, and, although I barely passed physical education, I represented Canada on the Olympic Team in speed skating.

It's fairly common to count up hurts, especially when you've had a lot of them. But this coping mechanism is as universally ineffective as it is common. So is bargaining. I went through a classic stage of bargaining a few years ago, when my hair started falling out again. I had been completely bald for many years and wore a wig much of that time. But for twenty-five years, the alopecia had gone into remission. As my hair started falling out again, my childhood nightmare returned, and I could hear the voices calling, "Baldy, Baldy." I was determined not to relive that part of my past. So I started bargaining. I asked myself one question: "What is the most important thing in the world to me, and will I give that up for my hair?" My waterfront retreat . . . could I give it up, just for hair? YES. I was struck by the immense importance of hair, the power it has, the power we give it.

I do not think my experiences are unique. Quite the contrary—they will probably resonate with most people who have chronic alopecia areata. With the diagnosis of alopecia areata, I became different from every other child I knew. I was forced to take "the road less traveled." Since that day, I have always chosen the less-traveled route; it now forms part of my philosophy of life. Effective coping involves constructing a philosophy of life that works. Fortunately for me, I was a pretty good athlete and, as my father had been instrumental in reviving the speed skating movement, speed skating naturally became my sport of choice.

We lived in Winnipeg, one of the coldest, windiest prairie cities in North America, and I learned to skate at the age of two. The community rink was right across the road from our home. By the age of seven, I was the fastest kid in our school. As the years went by, I developed the identity of a super athlete. It didn't matter how fast I could run or skate, though—it was never fast enough to escape the teasing and the torment. Nevertheless, my will to succeed in athletics served a purpose by helping me survive. In a sense, excelling in sports saved me, at least for a while.

Experiencing hair loss can affect our perception of everything in life. We can be prisoners of the way we think, and our perceptions can create a way of thinking that is often negative and unhelpful. Everywhere we turn, we can see the world through bald eyes, and we can learn to laugh or cry. As I looked up at the roof of my house last spring, I noticed some shingles missing; they reminded me of bald patches. My roof looked bad on the outside, and the missing shingles could cause problems. If the roof leaks, the plaster can erode. Putting shingles on the roof fixes the inside. But putting a wig on the head doesn't necessarily fix the inside. People need a different kind of renovation. We can renovate the inside by learning coping strategies.

We can learn to turn a negative perception around. We can start to see the lightness rather than the darkness. That's what coping is all about—turning the challenge into something positive. Bald eagles used to remind me of baldness. Now when I watch them soar, I see what they really stand for: strength and freedom.

Another reason Dr. Shapiro and I wrote this book is

because we have a bond with everyone who has alopecia areata: one by virtue of professional experience and the other by personal experience with the disease. Our different perspectives combine well to give us an understanding of the world of alopecia areata. That said, we also know that no two people with alopecia areata are alike. The material in this book is intended to be helpful and hopeful. Some sections may not apply to everyone: each person has to cope with alopecia areata in an individual way. The information that follows is there for you to explore, to sift and sort through; take from it what you need.

WENDY THOMPSON, M.A.

Acknowledgments

Many people supported the production of this book from conception to completion. First, we want to thank the Johns Hopkins University Press for providing professional guidance throughout the process and, in particular, Jacqueline Wehmueller, who brought to this project a sensitivity and gentle wisdom that are as critical to the editing process as they are to the disease. Our deeply felt thanks to Nina MacDonald, R.N. B.Sc.N., whose intelligence, expertise, and warmth has helped to make the University of British Columbia Hair Clinic a friendly, caring place for all alopecia areata patients.

I would like to acknowledge those who gave generously of their time and their talent, supporting me in a unique way—thus helping me to write the book while at the same time growing hair. To my dear friend Nancy Moore, who was with me every step of the way and who shared my excitement from acceptance through to completion. She read the manuscript countless times, applauding what read well and catching many details that needed work; she literally supported me through "thick and thin." To my gerontology colleague and friend, Sandra Cusack, Ph.D., for the hours of collaboration, creative writing assistance, and computer wizardry. More important, for her consis-

tently positive support and unfailing strength—there is no
one I would rather work with. To Gisèle Touzin, with
whom I have laughed and walked many miles—healing
and growing—thank you, my friend. To my late parents,
for teaching me that excellence is the minimum standard
and that, through adversity, we can become the best we
can be.

I also want to acknowledge others who were there for
me from the beginning. I am indebted to Susan N. Terkel
for all her help. Nan Dickie and Kristen McCahon, in
keeping with my Olympic spirit, created the working title
of this book, "Heads, You Win." Moyra Jones read the
first draft from cover to cover, responding enthusiastically
with helpful suggestions and the assurance that she was
there whenever I needed her. Sheila Jacobs provided valuable assistance in researching and writing. My hair dresser,
Euniris Yeung, adjusted her fee according to the amount
of hair I had. (It got down to ten bucks.) Joy Barkwill and
Lesley Cole offered daily personal and professional support in my workplace. Thank you all.

Finally, what a medical team I had. I wish to pay trib-
ute to Jerry Shapiro, M.D., my dermatologist and co-
author, whose leading-edge research and treatments gave
me direct access to the latest medical information and most
effective medical interventions. Saul Pilar, B.A.Sc., M.D.,
specialist in applying clinical psychoneuroimmunology
and nutrition, whose approach to medicine helped keep
my body, mind, and soul together throughout exhausting
treatment protocols, thank you for never giving up on me:
I am deeply grateful.

WENDY THOMPSON, M.A.

I would like to acknowledge and give special thanks to my initial mentor in dermatology, the late Dr. William Stewart, for encouraging me to enter the field of "Hair," Dr. David McLean for encouraging our University of British Columbia Hair Clinic to grow and flourish, and Dr. Harvey Lui and Dr. Stuart Maddin for their valuable practical insights on many "hair issues."

A special thanks to Dr. Vera Price and Dr. Wilma Bergfeld for allowing me to visit their hair clinics and learn from their great knowledge base.

I would also like to thank my parents—my late mother, Brajna, and my father, Philip—for instilling in me the desire to learn all I can and to do the best I could in any academic endeavor.

Another important thank you to my co-author, Wendy Thompson, for getting this project going. Her tenacity and creativity made it all possible.

A final thank you to all my alopecia areata patients, who have given me the privilege to be their "alopecia doctor." They have been an inspiration to me, and it has been an honor to be their doctor.

JERRY SHAPIRO, M.D.

Alopecia Areata

Understanding Alopecia Areata

Alopecia areata is an unpredictable and capricious medical condition that is not easy to pronounce (al-oh-*pee*-sheeah air-ee-*ah*-tah) and is anything but easy to live with. It is, however, a relatively common condition: more than two and a half million people in the United States and Canada have lost hair because of alopecia areata. Researchers say that 1.7 people in a hundred (or seventeen in a thousand) will experience this mysterious disorder by the time they reach the age of fifty.

In simplest terms alopecia areata may be described as a noncontagious disease that causes hair to fall out, generally in round patches. The word *alopecia* comes from the Greek word *alōpekia* and means "loss of hair," while *areata,* derived from the Latin, means "occurring in patches." Researchers and physicians don't yet know what causes alopecia areata, but they have learned a great deal about what controls hair growth. And they continue to do research with the goal of developing more effective treatments—and, someday, a cure—for alopecia areata.

There's no way to predict who might get alopecia areata. Alopecia areata is as likely to develop in females as in males, and it can occur at any age, although about 60 percent of people with alopecia areata develop the disorder before age twenty. There don't appear to be any cultural predispositions to the disorder, either. People all around the world have been affected.

Alopecia areata is also unpredictable in how it progresses in people who develop the condition. Some people who lose hair due to alopecia areata find that their hair regrows spontaneously in a relatively short time, while for others the condition goes on a steady course, and they continue to have patchy bald spots. The vast majority of people (approximately 90 percent) with alopecia areata will not lose all their hair: they will have bald patches that come and go. Some people, however, will lose all the hair on their scalp, or all the hair on their entire head and body. Different terms are used for these different patterns of hair loss. *Alopecia areata,* as noted above, is the term used to describe patchy hair loss, wherever on the body it occurs; *alopecia totalis* is the term used when a person loses all of his or her scalp hair; and *alopecia universalis* is used to describe the loss of all hair from the body.

People with alopecia areata, totalis, or universalis are usually otherwise perfectly healthy. For this reason the condition is considered to be medically benign. Still, few people would deny that having alopecia areata changes their lives. So, yes, in the physical sense, alopecia areata is a harmless condition. But psychologically, it is very painful. Call it what you will—patchy hair, baldness, or alopecia—hair loss is a complex problem causing both emotional and social trauma for millions of men, women, and children. It affects almost every aspect of their lives.

Most people, even people with alopecia, would agree that there are many worse conditions to have than hair loss. But most people would also agree that hair loss can cause inner turmoil, and that it can have an effect on social situations and personal interactions. In our culture, hair is seen as a symbol of vitality, a sign of style, and an integral part of beauty. How we wear our hair helps to define who we are, to ourselves as well as to other people. In such a culture the loss of hair can profoundly affect a person's quality of life.

Often, it's how *other* people react that is the most crucial factor in how well we cope. Whenever someone says "It's only hair" or "Hair loss is only a cosmetic problem" or "Just get a wig," you can be sure that they don't understand what it's like to lose hair. Losing hair can be devastating.

Because alopecia areata affects people's lives so dramatically, many people with alopecia areata will do almost anything to grow hair. They try various treatments and may experience a thousand times over the frustration that researchers feel over the lack of complete understanding of the condition and the lack of a cure. For these people, the loss of hair is so traumatic that growing hair becomes the focus of their lives. For others, the most important issue is different. They mainly want to look normal, and they find that wearing a hairpiece accomplishes that.

For children, the loss or lack of hair often becomes linked with their identity. Little girls with alopecia areata "don't look like little girls," and that is confusing for them. In adults, when self-concept and identity have already been formed, it is often a matter of discovering a new person— one who, in some instances, doesn't even resemble their former self.

Adults and children with alopecia areata initially experience a sense of profound loss. When we lose our hair, we also lose confidence, self-esteem, and sometimes even friends and partners. These losses erode the sense of who we are, and who we are is the essence of a meaningful life. In other words, we lose our identity. One man with alopecia totalis said, "When I look in the mirror, I don't recognize myself anymore. I don't know who that person is in the mirror looking back at me." A woman said, "When I lost my hair, I lost myself. I need to find me again." An adult who lost her hair as a child said, "I didn't lose myself. I never found myself."

Hair loss causes many people to search within themselves for a self-definition that is not so dependent on external appearance. They get beyond their discomfort and discontent and in the process become more of a "whole person." Despite what our culture tells us, it *is* possible to disregard the external and become focused on what goes on inside. And it *is* what goes on inside a person that really matters.

Alopecia areata strips people of much more than their physical appearance; it also takes away, at least for a while, their sense of well-being. Some idea of how profoundly this condition affects people is conveyed in the words of a person *with* hair who had been sexually abused. After viewing a documentary on alopecia areata, this person commented that alopecia areata was almost the same as sexual abuse and child abuse—you live with it every minute and every day of your life.

People who experience hair loss also experience an ongoing state of anxiety, because one of the significant characteristics of alopecia areata is that a person has no control over it (without medical intervention). It's not as though the person can go out and jog his or her way to healthy hair. The practicalities of wearing and maintaining a wig, painting on eyebrows (as many women do), or finding the right headgear (as many children do) is what we call the "outer" work of alopecia areata. This work takes time—lots of time—and emotional energy—lots of it.

Even so, the more difficult work is the "inner" work, which involves coming to terms with the loss or change of identity and self-esteem, and coping with the fear. Working toward acceptance, while at the same time never giving up on growing hair, is very difficult. Ashely Siegel, cofounder of the National Alopecia Areata Foundation (NAAF), writes about her experience coming to terms with this condition:

> The effect alopecia areata seems to have on people is to wipe out their self-esteem in a matter of moments. The whole ordeal from the dermatologist's office to the wig salon is often one degrading experience after another. Feeling so helpless and vulnerable, we wander around "inside out" for a time until we can put the pieces together again. I pushed people away for years. I missed out on feeling good and having great relationships for too long.
>
> I was afraid of the wind, of sex, of having people stand too close to my face (I was sure they were noticing my wig lines). I suspected that everyone told their friends about me and when I passed them on the street they said, "Oh, there's Ashely Siegel, the one with no

hair." I know children have a rough time with this. I hear stories about how they get teased at school. It does get better. As adults, I can tell you people are so hung up in their own concerns that your hair is the last on their list of obsessions. It's just your own list of obsessions that makes you crazy. I promise you that people are much too preoccupied with their own problems to dwell on yours.

It's funny, but as my friend Stephen says, "It's who you bring to the party that counts." Do you bring your alopecia areata? Do you bring your missing front tooth? Do you bring your speech impediment? I can choose to bring the truth about me—that I'm far greater than my alopecia areata. My little bald head is not who I am at all. (NAAF Newsletter no. 41, September/October 1989)

Ashely Siegel is right, in that what we look like is not who we are. In this society, however, people usually do judge a book by its cover, and so there's no denying that our looks affect our lives. It's hard to like who you are inside when you dislike who you are outside. Hair is one of the most important parts of how we look, and how we look is an important *part* of who we are. Any significant change in our appearance can greatly affect the feelings we have about ourselves.

Most men and women with alopecia areata say they are consumed by their baldness from the moment they wake up in the morning. With the first glance in the mirror, they begin to create their "masks." They look in every store window to make sure that their hair spray is still holding. They make sure there is a comb in every corner of their world.

Bald men get teased. Many feel self-conscious and less attractive, and they worry about their sex appeal. The same holds for women, who say that when they lose their hair, they feel as if they have lost their femininity. They, too, feel unattractive, and they worry that their partners will look elsewhere. Men, women, and children with alopecia areata, totalis, or universalis say that they feel extremely vulnerable and uncertain, and they're afraid that they will never be loved.

Clearly, chronic severe alopecia areata is a difficult condition, and it takes a lot of time and effort to adjust to it. Some people who have lost all their hair and have adjusted to wearing a hairpiece say that their worst fear is that their hair will grow back, because then they will have to go through the experience—the physical and emotional loss—again. They would rather *not* have their hair grow back.

Psychologists say every aspect of our self-image is tied to our hair. When people are robbed of their hair, their self-image is destroyed. It doesn't matter how many times we are told that having alopecia areata has built our strong character, or that we are more empathetic, or that we have a beautiful or handsome face or a good personality and that our hair loss doesn't matter. For most of us, it *does* matter. We are reminded daily of the significance of a beautiful head of hair and, in comparison, we feel insignificant. Society and the media make us feel inadequate and unappealing. We feel incomplete on the outside and empty on the inside. Hair can be a fashion statement, a signature; it can define our individuality; it can help us conform; it can defy authority; it can seduce; and it can fall out.

Our sense of certainty about who we are creates a comforting, secure, and constant feeling. This certainty is foundational to one's mental health. People who lose their hair have no choice. When choices are lost, our sense of certainty is lost, and so is a sense of control. When control is lost, so is our confidence and self-esteem. In a very real sense, our life is threatened—the life we "used" to have has changed.

Loss and Grieving

If you have never lost your hair, you have to work hard to imagine what it's like. Understanding baldness is very difficult unless you are or have been bald, because loss of hair is different from other losses. With sudden hair loss or slow patchy hair loss or slow diffuse hair loss, people look different, and they feel different on the inside. And when you feel different on the inside, you act different on the outside, although sometimes you're not even aware of it.

People look at other kinds of losses or handicaps through different lenses. Seeing someone in a wheelchair is a normal occurrence, and when people see someone in a wheelchair, they're likely to feel empathy and to want to help. A leg prosthesis is viewed differently from a hair prosthesis (i.e., a wig or toupee). A person sees a cast on someone's arm and asks what happened. A person sees bald patches or very thin hair on someone, on the other hand,

and stares but seldom asks what's wrong and may think that the person has cancer or something contagious, like leprosy. The point is that many illnesses or handicaps are more acceptable than baldness. In the hierarchy of disease processes or health conditions, hair loss is grossly misunderstood. Even people who have lost two or three fingers say they would rather lose a finger than lose their hair.

There is no disputing the fact that a life-threatening illness brings us up short: it changes our values, our outlook, our entire life. Believe it or not, that's the way it is with baldness. Balding indicates the loss of bodily function even if it is only the loss of a mere hair follicle. And even though hair loss is physically benign, coping mechanisms for surviving the psychological impact of hair loss are as critical as those for surviving any serious disease. In fact, many patients having chemotherapy say that the worst part of that treatment is losing their hair. Some people with cancer refuse to have chemotherapy so they won't lose their hair.

The emotional stages of having alopecia areata and other types of hair loss sometimes follow the stages of adjusting to terminal illness and death of a loved one described by Elisabeth Kübler-Ross. People go through some or all of these stages of loss and grieving: denial, anger, depression, bargaining, and acceptance. As with loss of any kind, a person with alopecia areata must work through each of these stages before reaching the final stage, acceptance. For some people the first step in coping is to read Kübler-Ross's book *On Death and Dying*. That helps them make sense of their feelings.

The stages of loss and grieving are critical concepts to understand when facing alopecia. Most of us associate grief with death—the ultimate loss. Throughout our lives we experience losses, some large some small. The major losses usually change us and often alter the course of our lives. In a very real sense, alopecia areata is a double loss. It is an external, life-changing loss that is visible to everyone, but it is also an internal loss. We lose our former self.

The first feeling experienced by people who have alopecia areata is a profound sense of loss that hurts them emotionally. This emotional pain causes them to grieve, a process that in turn enables them to work through the loss. Grieving our losses enables us to accept the changes that we need to face. While we are grieving, our emotional life may be unpredictable and unstable, as unpredictable and unstable as the alopecia is. We can never return to who we were before the loss, and even when our hair grows back, we will never forget.

What Next?

We acknowledge that hair is important and that we have no control over our hair loss. Where do we go from here? We learn to cope in a way that works for us. Ultimately, it is how well we cope that makes the difference. In *Man's Search for Meaning,* Viktor Frankl wrote, "What was really needed was a fundamental change in our attitude toward life. . . . It did not really matter what we expected from life, but rather what life expected from us."

First, remain hopeful. Martin Luther King Jr. wrote, "Everything that is done in the world is done by hope."

Hopeful people can work through the grief that comes with losing their hair. Frankly, often this is not a pleasant journey, and it is not one that many people would take willingly. It may involve the painful process of letting go of a self-concept that we have developed over time, perhaps since birth. It means redefining who we are now and in the future. Those who can simultaneously accept the challenge that hair loss presents and remain hopeful will probably work through their grief most successfully.

"Hope ever urges us on and tells us tomorrow will be better," said Albius Tibullus. Even people who have no hair can find hope in the fact that hair regrowth is a possibility. In people with alopecia areata, the hair follicles remain alive below the surface of the skin and are capable of growing hair at any time. The medical and scientific communities do not yet know the cause of alopecia areata; nor do we know why in some people hair begins to regrow. In life, however, and in nature—in the entire universe—there are many things we don't know. As Robert Fulghum noted in his book *It Was on Fire When I Lay Down on It*, "We don't know how water moves from the ground up through the trunk and out to the leaves of a tree." And we don't know how homing pigeons come home, how to cure the common cold, or why people lose and regrow hair. For everyone who is affected by alopecia areata, what we do know is that we need to learn more about this disease.

It is a difficult thing, trying to remain hopeful while at the same time accepting ourselves. When we truly accept ourselves, we have a different presence and people treat us better. When we move to a position of self-acceptance, we can begin to live life as the person we want to be. Hopeful people living with alopecia areata can learn to face hair loss rather than avoiding it, and begin to develop a new sense of self. "Healing is a matter of time, but it is sometimes also a matter of opportunity": so wrote the great humanist physician Hippocrates.

The Powerful History of Hair

Throughout history, hair has symbolized strength. Perhaps the best known example is the biblical story of Samson. When Delilah cut off all his hair, Samson lost his great strength and was captured by the Philistines. With the return of his hair came his renewed strength which allowed him to pull down the temple and destroy his enemies. "If I be shaved, then my strength will leave me, and I shall become weak, and be like any other man" (Judges 16:17).

Native warriors believed that when you scalped the enemy you would possess his strength and courage. The warrior with the greatest number of scalps was the most powerful.

One dramatic experience of a military recruit is to have his head shaved. The armed services believe that they can build character by creating bald men who all look alike, lose their identity, and feel vulnerable. Hair has power. That's what makes the prospect of losing it so devastating.

Most people never consider how much power their hair has until they lose it. Understanding the significance hair has had through history may help us feel better about our hair condition. Others before us also put a premium on having hair. "Hair Facts," a brochure by the Canadian Dermatology Association (1992), gives the following short history of hair:

> Although we don't have any record of how our ancient ancestors wore their hair, we know that even in the earliest days of human civilization, hair was considered to be an important asset to appearance. For example, archaeologists have discovered hair ornaments dating as far back as the New Stone Age in 8000 B.C.
>
> In ancient Egypt, men and women shaved their heads as a means of keeping their scalps scrupulously clean, and of keeping cool. To compensate for their lack of locks, they often wore braided wigs. In ancient Greece and Rome, many people wore hairbands to keep their hair neatly in place, often dusting their hair with gold dust. Bleached hair was in vogue in these cultures, and women often braided or curled their hair into elaborate styles. Altering the natural color of the hair was also the custom among the early Germanic peoples. The Angles and Saxons dyed their hair blue, green, and orange, while the Gauls colored theirs bright red.
>
> During the Middle Ages, men wore medium-length hair and unmarried women wore theirs loose. Married women traditionally covered their hair with a veil. Receding hairlines, routinely plucked that way with tweezers, were highly fashionable. By the 1600s, men had developed a preference for wearing their hair long, often in the form of flowing curls. Full, curly wigs called periwigs were very popular. Women often wore their hair piled high on their heads.

During the 1700s, very elaborate hairstyles became popular among both men and women. Women's hairstyles often had to be supported by small cushions and wire frames, and sleeping upright was a necessity. Bathing was only an occasional activity and hygiene was generally poor, so women carried small picks which they used to relieve the scalp itch caused by head lice. By the time the nineteenth century rolled around, hairstyles had become simple again. Women usually wore braids or topknots, while men slicked their short hair back with Macassar oil. (The chairback protectors known as antimacassars originated during this era.)

During the early 1900s, the permanent wave was invented. By the 1940s, it had been almost perfected and many women wore their hair in a short "bob" cut that was waved with permanent. The full look became fashionable in the 1950s, the beehive hairdos often accomplished by backcombing or teasing the hair. Needless to say, the hair was often severely damaged by this process. Perhaps in response to this, the 1960s and 1970s heralded the natural unisex look with long, straight hair the vogue for both men and women. This contrasted sharply with the 1950s fashion of crewcuts for men. The Afro style was also fashionable during these years.

During the 1980s, most people opted for natural-looking hairstyles, and variety was "in," as people personalized their looks through state-of-the-art haircoloring, highlighting, waving, and straightening techniques. Shampoo and conditioner formulas were developed that were much better for hair than the old-fashioned harsh treatments.

By this time there had been a significant shift in public thinking that placed science and medicine squarely in
the hair care picture. A dermatologist was just as likely
to be consulted for a hair problem as a beautician. And
so on, to the next century, for even more advances in
hair care. Already on the horizon is a laser-emitting
comb that lightens hair by destroying the pigment within. There will almost certainly be better treatments for
baldness, as more and more aging baby boomers seek
help for hair loss.

Hair is part of our self-definition. Hair is powerful.
Preoccupation with hair has been a consistent feature of
human societies through the ages. And alopecia areata is
a condition that challenges the best of us.

Coping with Hair Loss

Many people have written books about their personal experiences with an illness. They often begin their stories with a description of when and where they first learned the name of their disease or disorder, who told them, and how the news was given. Almost every single one of these authors—even those who were prepared for this news, because they suspected it or because their doctor had prepared them for it—say that their first reaction was one of shock or disbelief. They want to cover their ears or run out of the doctor's office, or they tell the doctor that something must be wrong with the diagnosis. When you think about it, it's hard to imagine how anyone could be prepared to be told that he or she has a disease or disorder that could profoundly affect life from this moment on.

Just hearing the name of the disease can throw people into a crisis, but learning how that disease or disorder will affect them can be overwhelming and, sometimes, devastating. Only people whose health is less than perfect can fully understand the meaning of the expression "If you've got your health, you've got everything."

Most people who are diagnosed with alopecia areata have never heard of it. The sound of the words is as foreign as the disease itself. After learning that their hair loss is caused by alopecia areata, they learn that there is no cure for this poorly understood disorder.

For most people, alopecia affects them emotionally more than physically or socially. Beginning from when they first notice that they are losing hair, then through the process of being diagnosed, going through treatments, and adjusting to having a new appearance, people experience a multitude of emotions, ranging from disbelief to fear, sadness to anger, and shame to alienation.

Alopecia areata also causes emotional changes in the family and friends of the person affected. People many times feel sad over the loss of their loved one as he or she was, as he or she used to look. Spouses and other partners, and siblings and other family members, may feel ashamed of the person with alopecia areata and may resent him or her, and perhaps even be angry at the person for having made them feel socially conspicuous.

Parents often feel guilty, wondering whether they may have genetically contributed to their child's disease, and helplessly frustrated because they cannot stop the disease and ease their child's emotional pain. They may also develop fears about their child's health, worrying that some other apparently random health hazard is in store for their child, perhaps something more menacing, something else for which they aren't prepared and for which there is no cure.

People with alopecia areata are unhappy about the way they look, and they feel conspicuous. Having other people stare and say unkind things, of course, only makes it more difficult for people with alopecia areata to cope. Most people who don't have alopecia areata or who don't know someone with the condition don't understand it, and they're likely to say something stupid simply because they don't understand. Their comments may be related to their mistaken belief that only someone who is very sick would have little or no hair. There's also a lot of plain and simple prejudice in the world against anyone who doesn't look exactly "normal."

Hair Loss Is a Life-Changing Event

Life for people with alopecia areata is full of stresses and strains. People who describe how their lives have changed because of hair loss say:

- I look strange. I get sad and frustrated.
- It's like experiencing death, like grief.
- It really limited job prospects for the future.
- I'm living more for the moment. Everything seems much more precious.
- I think twice before going swimming or running.

They say that the worst things about losing hair are:

- The hassle of wearing a wig every day
- The constant worry about appearance, about whether others will notice their hair loss or their wig
- Fear that they might go completely bald
- Trying to hide their hair loss from people
- Losing self-esteem and trying to get it back and maintain it
- Losing eyebrows and eyelashes
- Not being able to feel natural
- Wondering if they will have to deal with this forever

People who have been living with hair loss for a while say that they have gained some things because of their hair loss:

- I'm stronger. More independent, less insecure.
- I'm more optimistic.
- I have inner strength and inner peace.
- I have a better appreciation of others and especially a better insight into other people's disabilities.
- I've learned not to feel sorry for myself and to get on with life.
- I don't judge other people by their appearance any more.

People with alopecia sometimes think that there is something wrong with them because they have such a wide range of feelings, and because those feelings are so intense. As the above statements make clear, however, reactions to hair loss vary widely. Different people react to hair loss in different ways. Thinking that there's something wrong with you because of what you're feeling only adds to your burden. It's important to acknowledge that losing hair is something that makes people feel different from how they felt before. People react to hair loss, and they react to having a disorder that can't be cured and that affects them so profoundly. That's only normal.

Some emotions are private, such as feelings of sadness, loss, or hopelessness. A person who feels hopeless usually is afraid about what the future holds. People may also blame themselves for somehow bringing the disease on themselves, and they feel guilty about that. People feel frustrated about the lack of control they have over it and the lack of medical progress in understanding it. They are angry because it's an "unfair" disease—no one knows why it strikes one person and not another. "Why me?" is a question many people with alopecia have asked themselves.

Many people suffer in silence, feeling isolated from the people around them, who don't understand. A sense of isolation is a common feeling for someone with alopecia areata. Sometimes people withdraw socially and then feel isolated; sometimes people begin to feel isolated and then withdraw socially. People with alopecia may feel that other people are ignoring them, or they may be concerned that other people keep staring at them. They may think that no one really understands their hair loss—or them. Their lifestyle may change dramatically. They may give up most of their former activities and only do things that make them feel safe—often times precious few for someone wearing a wig.

One of the surprisingly strong emotions alopecia areata can produce in many people is feeling out of control. People with alopecia areata don't know what causes their condition or how long it will last, and there are no treatments that are guaranteed to initiate hair growth. When people have a disease that is out of their control, and out of their doctor's control, the resulting sense of helplessness may cause depression. Many people with hair loss feel depressed when they compare their present situation to the way things were. Some find that their moods swing more, and more easily. If you are someone who has been depressed before, you may find that you recognize some aspects of your response to hair loss. If you have seldom been down in the past, you may find that depression is a frightening new emotion.

At first, many people with alopecia experience a drop in self-esteem, and some people even feel self-loathing. People worry that others will not love them now that they have lost hair. Many people have difficulties with their partner or family, and their sex life may change. These feelings come about because of their concern over how other people will respond to them. They're afraid that other people will find out that they have the disease, or will discover that they wear a wig; they may be afraid that they will be verbally or even physically abused. Everyone with alopecia areata has had to cope with embarrassment that may at times be acute.

The various emotions that people with alopecia areata experience may cause them to become withdrawn and isolated, at work, at home, and socially. They may even withdraw from their family because they feel guilty for everything that their hair loss is putting their loved ones through. They may try to cope by going to an extreme of one sort or another—searching relentlessly for an answer or a cure for the disease to the exclusion of all else in life, or turning to drink or drugs—or religion—in a big way.

There are more effective ways to cope. This chapter describes various coping skills as well as some ways to think about things in a slightly different light. Some of these strategies will be new to you. We suggest that you read through this chapter with an open mind—you never know when one of these strategies will be the one you need most. We realize that not all of the ideas in this chapter will be useful for every person, however. The idea is to choose the techniques that appeal to you, and use them to change your perspective so that, over time, you can cope better with the demands that alopecia areata places on you.

Determining Your Personal Style of Coping

Personal coping styles vary widely: one person may cope by using denial—adopting the philosophy that if he or she ignores the problem it will go away—another by being analytical and seeking information. Some people cope best by "getting it out"—by crying or finding someone to confide in, or by praying or meditating. If you haven't done so before, now is the time to think about your own coping style.

Think about how you generally cope. Are you calm or do you get nervous when faced with a crisis? Are you still and quiet, or do you pace and chatter? When you're trying to solve a problem, are you persistent, or do you give up easily?

Take some time to remember how you handled trouble before the alopecia areata was diagnosed—not just the crises that seemed overwhelming, but also the smaller problems that you handled well. What contributed to your success? Then think about how you can apply your strengths to this new challenge, the challenge of hair loss.

Make sure to give your body the best chance to deal with this condition. That means getting enough sleep, eating good, wholesome food and supplements if needed, getting regular physical exercise, and managing stress levels.

Consider your emotional life. How "in touch" with your feelings are you? You may find it easy, or you may find it difficult, to express your emotions. How have you coped in the past with anger? With fear? With depression? With guilt? These are some of the feelings people commonly experience along with hair loss.

Think about how important control is to you in your life. Because they can't control their condition, people with alopecia areata often discover the value of letting go of what they cannot control. They discover the lessons of the serenity prayer: "God, grant me the serenity to accept the things I cannot change, the courage to change the things I can, and the wisdom to know the difference." Or they develop a new sense of control, one that comes from what they *make of* the experience. They realize that they can change the way they feel about something by reframing it in a more positive way.

People are not born copers, but coping skills and perspectives are devices that anyone can pick up and apply to life. And once they learn to cope, people with alopecia areata find that they're no longer as anxious, at least in part because they aren't focused on themselves all the time. They can relax a bit about their condition and about other people's reaction to it, and begin again to take an active part in the world around them.

Most people take a long time to adapt to change, especially to a sudden and unexpected change like alopecia areata. Give yourself time, and don't expect too much of yourself all at once. Try to be hopeful. Be kind to yourself.

As one person in our support group said, "We need to be allowed to be weak every once in a while. We need a break from being strong and courageous." A certain amount of denial is okay. Try to take things one at a time.

Many people who have experienced loss and trauma find it helpful to talk with a mental health professional who can help them work through their feelings and learn coping skills. Although it is common for people with alopecia areata to experience a variety of psychological reactions, if your feelings are intense and if you feel overwhelmed by them, or if your feelings and reactions are persistent, you should give counseling a try. Also, if you no longer participate in activities that used to bring joy to your life, if you find yourself missing work or school frequently, or if you no longer feel you can talk to or reach out to those who are close to you, you should consider counseling.

We highly recommend alopecia areata support groups, and often these groups alone provide sufficient help. However, obtaining counseling from a trained professional can be beneficial as well. Counseling gives you more time to focus on your own specific experiences, and provides a safe environment to share your feelings knowing that what you say will be kept in the strictest confidence. This knowledge may help you discuss issues that you may not want to share in front of a group.

To find a mental health professional, you can ask your physician for a referral, call your local mental health association for a recommendation, ask your friends if they can recommend someone, or contact the National Alopecia Are-

ata Foundation's Mental Health Committee, which may
be able to refer you to someone in your area. When you
ask for a referral or a recommendation, be sure to say that
you're seeking help in coping with a physical loss, since
there are psychologists, social workers, and other coun-
selors who specialize in helping people with this kind of
challenge.

Coping by Getting the Facts

We discuss medical treatments in the next chapter, but
if you've been diagnosed with alopecia areata you probably already know that there is no cure yet, and that the
currently available medical treatments aren't effective for
everyone. It's possible that you will grow your hair back,
and it's possible that you won't be able to grow your hair
back. One way to cope, though, is to learn about the
disease.

As we acknowledged earlier, some people cope by becoming informed, while others prefer not to know much
or anything about their illness. These represent different
styles of coping. You should seek out as much information as you want to have.

For most people, the more they understand, the more
in control they feel. One advantage of becoming informed
is that you will feel more confident when you talk with
medical professionals. Also, the information will give you
a focus, so that you don't feel lost in the strange new
world of hair loss.

One excellent source of information is the National Alopecia Areata Foundation (NAAF), which was founded in

1981 by Ashely Siegel and dermatologist Dr. Vera Price. Ashely Siegel had the disease and was looking both for help and for other people with alopecia areata with whom she could share her problems and concerns. NAAF has grown into an international center of alopecia areata information and service. The foundation is governed by a volunteer board of directors and has a professional executive director.

NAAF raises money to sponsor a variety of programs designed to benefit people with alopecia areata. Funds provided by the foundation sponsor research on causes, effective treatments, and, eventually, a cure; service to those with the disease; education of representatives of federal and state governments concerning the need for fairer insurance laws and greater government-sponsored research; and ongoing public awareness programs.

As part of its public awareness programs, the foundation disseminates information about alopecia areata through brochures placed in doctors' offices. It also publishes a newsletter and has developed a seven-minute videotape for children called *This Weird Thing That Makes My Hair Fall Out;* you can get a free copy by calling or writing NAAF. In addition, NAAF works hard to educate legislators regarding health care and other issues of concern to people with alopecia areata. Its executive director has testified before congressional committees.

The *National Alopecia Areata Foundation Newsletter,* which is published five times a year, provides a forum through which people with alopecia areata and their friends and families can interact and receive the latest information on all aspects of the disease. The newsletter makes it possible for those with alopecia areata to speak out about the challenges associated with the condition and to share ideas about how to deal with them. It contains news about research and treatments as well as innovative and tried-and-true cosmetic and wig tips. You can subscribe to the newsletter for a donation of $35, or whatever you can afford, by contacting the National Alopecia Areata Foundation (see Resources).

People from all over the world who have alopecia areata come together at the annual NAAF International Conference. People attending this three-day event are immersed in information about medical treatments, ongoing and new research, coping strategies, and progress in cosmetic and fashion techniques. You may wish to attend one of the NAAF conferences, or even make attending the conference an annual event. At the conference you'll be able to share with others who understand your feelings based on their firsthand experience. The intensity of the weekend will help you establish personal and emotional connections with other people that often result in long-lasting friendships. Nearly everyone who attends the conference says that it has a positive effect on their lives.

In addition to the National Alopecia Areata Foundation, there are other good sources of information about alopecia areata. We've already mentioned that other people with the disease can often provide information as well as support. So can your family physician and dermatologist. Joining or forming a support group as well as attending conferences and workshops can be very helpful.

Some hospitals or clinics will provide a place where support groups can meet, if there's enough interest in the community, and they may help to publicize the meetings, as well. Ask your doctor about this, or contact the public relations office of your community hospital for more information.

As part of your strategy of coping by becoming informed, you'll want to gather information about treatment options, including the effectiveness, cost, and side effects of each one. Ask questions. Become familiar with your particular pattern and symptoms. Keep a journal of your treatments: record what the treatment was, including the dose, if appropriate, how well it worked, how long it lasted, what the side effects were, and, when appropriate, why you discontinued it. Keep a record of your appointments with your doctor or doctors, so you'll be able to remember who made specific recommendations, and when.

The known is usually easier to cope with than the unknown. It is important to become familiar with each treatment and how it affects you. Not only does knowledge reduce fear, it helps us feel more in control. As noted earlier, one of the worst feelings experienced by people with alopecia areata is feeling out of control. Therefore anything we do that helps us feel in control will ultimately help us feel better.

Adjusting the Attitude

Beginning a treatment plan can be an empowering experience because there is hope that a treatment will work for you. But even exploring treatment options can give you a sense of hope. While there is no cure for alopecia areata, there are different treatments, and one of them may work for you. If one treatment is unsuccessful, there are others to try. That said, it's important to add that it's better to locate your hope in an internal source instead of in a particular treatment—that is, it's better to locate your hope in a source over which *you* have control. Your attitude, for example. Working on attitude gives you good backup strategies in case treatment isn't successful. Thus, whatever happens in the outside world or on your scalp, you will still have *you* to help you cope.

Remind yourself of what makes you happy, and keep a list to refresh your memory. The little things in life that are free and abundant can be every bit as pleasurable as something that costs money. Would you enjoy feeding birds over a picnic lunch in a park? Watching the sun rise or set from a peaceful vantage point? Taking your niece or nephew for a walk around the harbor? Keep a list of such activities, so you can refer to it if you need a reminder of the things that give you pleasure. Take time to think:

- What is most important in your life?
- What is your philosophy of life?
- What do you need? What do you want?
- What is your lifestyle? Is it outdoorsy? Fashion conscious? Intellectual?
- What would you like more of in your life: fun, vacations, time to read, a new kitchen?
- What would you like to have less of: stress, arguments, basement junk?

What changes can you make in your life that would help you have an overall attitude that would make it easier for you to cope with alopecia areata? Who might be able to help you with these changes? The aim is to keep a balance between doing what you can about your hair loss and not forgetting that you have a lot more going on in your life than just your hair. Talk to friends and others who have gone through loss, chronic illness, or disability. Don't just talk about yourself—ask about their experiences, and really listen to what they have to say.

Finally, doing a daily attitude check is a good idea. While you're checking your attitude, try to keep negative thoughts at bay. Focus on what's positive in your life and think about what you can do to increase the positives. You may have to take some risks in your life to make change. Taking risks, even if they are calculated risks, can be exciting and fun. And of course, there's nothing like having fun to help adjust the old attitude.

Controlling Stress

Having alopecia areata is often very stressful, but having a high level of stress in your life is not conducive to coping. To decrease your stress, first find out what your sources of stress are, and then start a stress management program. What's the most stressful thing for you about having alopecia areata? For some people, it's looking in the mirror every morning without hair. For others, not being able to answer the door without their wig on, or always having to wear a wig, causes major stress.

To deal with stress, you'll need to develop a stress management program. You can begin anywhere—with exercise, meditation, relaxation techniques—and then build from there. Exercise is part of every stress management program, because exercise is a natural way to release tension from the body and the mind. The positive effects of exercise are very useful in coping with hair loss. We can think more positively and are better able to combat stress, anxiety, and even depression, if we exercise. If you can exercise three to five times every week, you will feel much more relaxed and less stressed.

Daily prayer or meditation can provide stability and inner peace to help you balance whatever else is going on in your life. Concentrating on the spiritual side may help you put your physical loss into perspective. Another possibility is to learn a relaxation technique that works for you. Relaxing gives your mind and your body a break from everyday life and can refresh you for taking on new challenges.

You can learn to relax completely, through yoga or meditation, hypnosis or biofeedback. In a completely relaxed state we are most receptive to experiencing peace, love, warmth, "grounding," or "centering," and to using positive visualization to confront the disease process or accomplish other goals. Visualization is a technique used in spheres as diverse as sales training, sports training, and cancer therapy. People who visualize their goal very clearly seem to attain it more easily—whether it's the Porsche they're dying for, or holding up the football trophy to a cheering crowd.

Now more than ever you'll need to pamper your whole

self and give yourself the gift of time to pray or meditate or do yoga or whatever keeps you sane. Allow yourself to pamper your mind with entertaining fiction or theater or film. Take a trip, big or small, according to what your budget can stand; even a visit to relations or friends can give you a break from routine and provide a fresh outlook.

Accept yourself for who and where you are. Accept that you have down times, just like everyone. Remind yourself that it is okay to have "bad hair days." Acknowledge and respect yourself. Consider all that you have been through, in life and with your alopecia. Be proud of yourself, stand tall, and hold your head up; your feelings will follow your body language and actions.

Coping with Negative Thoughts and Feelings

When people with alopecia areata are asked, "What are your greatest fears about having lost or losing hair?" they say:

- How I'll look when it's all gone
- People making fun of me
- That I'll never have hair again
- That I'm not really well and may die
- That my partner will not find me attractive
- Having to wear a wig and having it fall off
- Being embarrassed

As noted earlier in this chapter, having fears and anxieties when you have alopecia areata is normal, but you still need to learn to cope with them, so you can reclaim your self-esteem, and your *self*. One very effective way to

cope with negative feelings is to make a pact with yourself about what you will and will not say to yourself.
Every time that you say or do anything, you are saying something about yourself to yourself. How you treat yourself
as a person with not much hair tells you what kind of person you think you are. One man, for example, stopped having a social life for a couple of years after his hair fell out;
later, he saw that he was sending himself the message that
he didn't deserve a social life, that being hairless meant he
was unacceptable as a friend or acquaintance. Actions,
thoughts, and statements affect the emotions and therefore
the body.

Learn to accent the positive in your thinking, your actions, your writing, your verbal communications. This is
a terrific attitude to develop for whatever life may bring.
Develop a positive philosophy about life. Think "I can"
instead of "I can't," and focus on the positive aspects of
yourself, your achievements in life, and all the good things
you have and do. Try to spend time with people who are
positive and encouraging. Set goals, however small, to give
yourself a sense of control and competence, to give yourself the message that you do just fine.

Don't stop at the mirror and dwell on your lack of hair.
Paste some positive phrases on your mirror so that, when
you are using the mirror, you'll read statements such as
"I'm going to create a great day for myself and others."

Here's another suggestion: Instead of worrying all day,
set aside time to worry about your hair loss, say, between
7:00 and 8:00 P.M. By postponing your worry time, you'll
free up your energy during the day for your work, and by

allowing yourself a full hour for worrying, you may quickly discover that you don't have worries enough to fill the time. You may find it difficult to worry for a full hour in the evening. You may even forget to keep the "anxiety" appointment.

Develop a habit, such as journal writing, that will make it easier for you to get through your day. Start working on it and soon it will be part of you. Log your thoughts, feelings, and questions. When you can look back on what you were thinking about some months or weeks or years earlier, you get a perspective on where you are now. You can congratulate yourself on your progress and achievements, and identify areas that need better focus or more effort.

Fill your life with things and activities you enjoy—but don't make it so full that you create more stress. Spend money on glittery ornaments for your wig, or on a manicure or quality makeup. Set up lunch dates with people whose company you really enjoy at a relaxing place where the food is good. Buy a small luxury item to make bath time a time of pampering—a scented candle or a herbal bath. Try the unexpected, a new experience, to give yourself a fresh perspective. If you normally treat yourself with ice cream or chocolate, this time buy yourself an expensive glossy magazine or beautiful art book from a secondhand bookstore. Have a weekend away in a most unlikely place—at a lakeside resort, if you are a big city lover, in a city museum or library, if your normal suburban weekend is filled with shopping, washing, and vacuuming. Buy yourself a kite and learn to fly it.

Getting busy with work is another great way to shake

the negative thoughts from your head. Do one thing each day that you can successfully finish. Also, set yourself longer-term goals, things to be accomplished by the end of a few days, a week, or a month, that have nothing to do with hair loss. Write them down and put them where you can see them. Make them specific, precise, and achievable. The aim is to reinforce your self-esteem and improve your life, not to leave you feeling like a failure for not accomplishing something—never mind regrowing hair. Be sure to reward yourself for your accomplishments.

Diana Ross sings about making this world a better place. It's a good motto for me. You may want to consider giving your time, self, and talents to others, or volunteering your services and helping someone less fortunate. Perhaps it's hard to find a cause that really turns you on, but you can probably figure out what it is for you. It could be as big as finding all the lonely senior citizens in your community and rounding up volunteers to visit them twice a week. It could be earning twice as much salary, so you have more to give to your family and friends. It could be volunteering at your community hospice program. It could be learning how to cook Mexican. Get passionate about something.

If a head full of hair is the only thing you're passionate about, you may want to consider starting a fund-raising campaign to raise money for research. (Have you seen the movie *Lorenzo's Oil*?) Another thing we can do is educate others about alopecia areata. Educating others teaches us about ourselves, helps others to understand us, and helps others who have alopecia areata, because more people understand. Try changing just a small corner of your world—for example, campaign to have your community swimming pool install private changing rooms. It's very difficult to take off your wig to put on a bathing cap or to be naked in front of others without normal body hair, and in particular no pubic hair.

Make contact with other people with alopecia areata. Helping others helps you. Join or start an alopecia areata support group. Motivate others to take action. Let your relatives, friends, and community resources know what your situation is and what they can do to help. Practice asking for help.

Building Relationships with Family and Friends

People cope better when they have a network of supportive friends and family members. It's important not to shut these people out when you develop alopecia areata, but to bring them even closer, by educating them about the disease and letting them know how it is affecting you. Describe the feelings you have that are associated with alopecia areata. Tell them:

- Some days I hate the way I look.
- I'd love to go swimming and not have to worry about my wig.
- I hate how itchy my head is.
- Some days I feel like a freak.

Then tell your family and friends what you need from them by way of support. Say:

- Give me a compliment once in a while.
- Acknowledge the courage that it takes to deal with this condition.
- Treat me as normal.
- Ask me to talk about it and listen to how it is and how it feels.
- Give me privacy to fix my wig and makeup.
- Tell me you love me.
- Be empathic and supportive and sensitive.
- Don't joke about it until I'm ready.

Encourage family sharing, understanding, and discussion of the disease. Take a family member with you when you go for a treatment, and share the experience, the questions, the feelings. Believe people when they tell you that you look good.

Family members may think you don't have a problem and that you're fussing too much about your hair loss. They won't necessarily understand the emotional impact of alopecia areata. They may think that you're under stress—You are!—and that you should "get your act together." You can't force everyone to understand, but a very important part of adjusting to this disease is for your family and friends to learn to adjust, as well. Make sure your family and friends are informed. Educate them: it's a good way of coping, and everyone will feel better.

Finally, surround yourself with people whose company you enjoy. If you thought someone was critical or negative before your hair fell out, you especially don't need to spend time with that person now, at a vulnerable time in your life. Think carefully about which of the people you know enhance your life, appreciate you, and make you feel positive about life and about yourself. Cultivate *them* as friends.

Alopecia and Sexuality

Not knowing how to deal with alopecia in a sexual relationship can be upsetting and confusing and frustrating, both emotionally and sexually. Sexual relationships, like all relationships, are a tangled combination of physical responses, conversational flirting or foreplay, energy level, self-confidence, relaxation, past emotional issues and responses, and, for some, a spiritual dimension. This is why people say that the most important sexual organ is between the ears, and why some physically unattractive people can be extremely sexy.

Because the emotional and mental aspects of a satisfying sexual relationship are as important as, if not more important than, physical attraction, it's not surprising that much of a person's sexual confidence rests on the inner concept of self-esteem. When hair loss has diminished self-esteem, a sexual encounter can increase anxiety and diminish confidence. People with alopecia areata or alopecia universalis often have to decide how much to reveal, and when in the course of a relationship to reveal it. The anxiety created by this situation makes the relaxation and enjoyment essential to a close sexual relationship difficult to attain.

One woman broke down when describing how emotionally exhausting she found dating because of her uncertainty about if and how to tell her date about her hair loss. A kiss was not a kiss for her; it was an exercise in tactical response designed to prevent her date's hand from stroking or kissing her "hair," her neck, or her face near the hairline. It's sad that this woman and her date are having such different, and confusing, experiences of a kiss, when they could be relating and communicating at a deeper level.

There is plenty of anthropological and sociological evidence to show that hair is frequently associated with sexiness, and in the last decade it seems as though the bigger the hair, the bigger the sex appeal. Luckily, this is a logical fallacy. Just because hair can be sexy, that doesn't mean that *only* hair is sexy. Remember that your personal qualities are a big part of your attraction for your partner. Make a list of the things that you find sexy about your date or would-be date, and then ask yourself how big a part his or her hair plays. Can you imagine finding your date sexy if his or her hair wasn't so hot? How about if hair wasn't in the equation? Advertising and movies push the notion that appearance—that is, what product you can buy to "improve" your appearance—is beauty. But in a culture bombarded with these images of impossibly thin, beautiful women and young, dashing hunks, it takes a cool head to figure out for yourself that appearance isn't the most important factor in a relationship.

What holds many people back is not the lack of head hair as much as sparse or absent body hair, especially pubic hair. One young man went for four years without dating, although he had plenty of friends, including some who showed definite sexual interest. He could joke with these women, even flirt, but when it came to anything more than touching an arm, or maybe seeing someone home who was obviously interested, he just froze. He couldn't bring himself to embark on a journey whose course looked scary, whose end was unknown. He longed for contact, but was worried he wouldn't know where to stop—and he was sure he would have to stop, because without his pubic hair he felt almost castrated, like a boy and not a man.

This sense of vulnerability is common to most men and women (and teenagers) who have less pubic hair than normal. It is understandable, given the physical delicacy of these very private parts of our bodies. But it's also a question of intimacy and trust—you want to know your partner will not burst out laughing, or run away screaming. Think of ways to increase your intimacy first, ways that have nothing to do with hair. Prepare steps on this journey. After all, if you do have a relationship with this person and some ill health or disability strikes, it's good to have some idea how he or she might react. Build up your relationship on a solid foundation.

As relationships progress, people with alopecia areata have reported that the challenges change. Many surmount the obstacles they encounter with courage and trust and optimism—they don't know for sure they can cope with this, but they'll try. As commitment grows between a couple, most have talked at length about the condition and experience of alopecia. They may spend time together without "hair." They may start to dream, to plan.

One woman with alopecia areata had a very loving

boyfriend who wanted to get married after dating for a few months. Her friends thought she was crazy for not accepting, but she felt too anxious about her hair. Would his family freak out? Would his father, something of a comedian, joke about it? How would she cope with all the stress of a wedding, and with the anxiety about her hairpiece as well? She imagined the dozens of humiliating, clownish, painful mishaps that might blight what should be the happiest day of her life. Her veil might get tangled up with her father's tuxedo buttons as he handed her over to her bridegroom—and pull her wig off with it. It might get caught on flowers or greenery, or on gift bows. It might get yanked by her playful four-year-old niece.

Or what if the couple had children who inherited their mother's hair loss? How would she cope with their trauma, with the guilt that she would feel? This woman had shown great courage in telling her boyfriend about her hair loss when they began to get close, but she balked at further intimacy: she felt it was enough for him to bear, having a girlfriend without hair, without burdening him with her worries. So she stayed cool and noncommittal, without explaining. Depending on the couple and the circumstances, a story such as this can have many different endings.

Some people might have difficulty understanding this woman's problem. But for most people with alopecia areata, it's not just a matter of putting on a hairpiece and forgetting about it. Wearing a hairpiece affects many aspects of everyday life, and many people—like the woman who was worried about her wedding day—live with a constant

low level of anxiety about whether it's on straight and
whether it might come off. This anxiety is understandably
heightened at the prospect of an intimate encounter. The
best advice here is the same advice that applies to anyone
who is considering becoming intimate with someone, and
that is to postpone physical intimacy until a relationship
of mutual trust and understanding has been established.

Humor

Some people can use humor to lighten things up. But
don't use humor to hide your feelings. For example, after
losing patches of hair, an eight-year-old boy became more
and more withdrawn at home, although he seemed to
cope well at school. In fact, his teacher complained that,
if anything, he was too boisterous. The boy denied that he
was having a problem, but after finding him crying one
day, his father talked with him and discovered that, in
order to deal with teasing and bullying at school, the boy
had turned into the class clown. He was always able to get
a joke in about his appearance first, to deflect hostility.
Other children in the class encouraged his clowning, but
the feelings of fear and hurt he hid beneath the jokes sur-
faced when he was safely at home, and made him feel
confused.

As long as it's not being used to mask our true feelings—even from ourselves—humor can be a very useful
way of coping. For example, it can defuse many situations. One bald woman introduced herself to people at a
meeting by briefly explaining alopecia areata and describing herself as "the one with the cool head." This intro-

duction helped other people both understand the condition and feel more comfortable with their colleague. They understood that she could "handle it."

As children, teenagers, and adults, we are faced with an infinite number of crises throughout our lives. If you have alopecia areata, the loss of hair may be the most difficult crisis that you will ever have to face. In Chinese characters, the symbol for crisis and opportunity are the same. If you can meet this crisis as an opportunity, an opportunity to develop who you are as a human being and to be the best you can be, you will be a winner.

Alopecia areata presents a great challenge to each of us who have it. You are only a "victim of alopecia areata" if you give up on yourself. Investing hope in the "inner you" guarantees rich rewards—strength of character, development of talents and skills, the opportunity to discover and claim yourself. Investing in the outer you is more tenuous, because the course of the disease is capricious and there is no cure at present. There are, however, treatments that are effective for some people some of the time, and there are treatments that work for some of the people almost all of the time. The more you know about them, the better your chances of topping up that new inner you with hair.

THREE

Diagnosis, Treatment, and the Latest Research

Alopecia areata is a disease that causes loss of hair on the scalp and sometimes elsewhere on the body. As we noted in chapter 1, alopecia areata is a relatively benign disease: it doesn't cause any permanent physical damage or physical pain, it is not contagious, and it is usually not a warning of any other disease. In most cases, the probability of regrowth is high, because the hair follicles—the small sacs on the scalp where individual hairs grow—are not permanently harmed when the hairs break off or fall out. Doctors and researchers don't fully understand this disease, but the thinking now is that it is most likely a kind of allergic reaction to one's own hair.

Often, all three types of alopecia—areata, totalis, and universalis—are referred to as *alopecia areata,* but the terms are designed to be used to distinguish between different patterns of hair loss. *Alopecia areata* refers to varying amounts of patchy hair loss, from one small bald patch to larger areas with little or no hair; this kind of hair loss generally takes place on the scalp, but any hair-bearing area on the body, such as the beard or the pubic area, may be affected. In *alopecia totalis,* all the hair on the scalp is lost, and the surface of the scalp becomes totally smooth. *Alopecia universalis* means loss of all hair on the head and the body, including eyelashes and eyebrows, underarm hair, and pubic hair. This form of the disease has some physical disadvantages. For example, people with alopecia universalis don't have any eyebrows, so they have to contend with perspiration trickling into their eyes; also, because they have no eyelashes, they have no protection from dust and glare. The lack of nose hair means their nostrils and sinuses have no protection from foreign particles in the air.

The other areas of the body that may be affected by this disease are the fingernails and toenails. One explanation for the involvement of the nails is that there are biological and chemical similarities between hair and nails— both are composed of dead protein, fed by a living base or root. People with alopecia may have changes in their fingernails and toenails such as pinprick indentations or ridges or roughness. In most cases, these changes in the nails can only be seen on close examination.

As anyone with alopecia areata knows, the biggest challenge presented by the disease is the challenge of coping emotionally. But the physical challenges of alopecia, from securing a wig in a way that provides some sense of confidence that it won't fall off, to keeping sweat out of your eyes during exercise or in a stressful situation, can also be a burden. And the social problems of alopecia range from teasing to loss of a job and divorce and everything in between, including being accused of belonging to an extremist cult because of your bald head. The total effect of the disease can be a sudden and sometimes long-lasting change in life, lifestyle, and even personality.

For a disease that has such a significant impact on your

life, it's important to find out everything that you can about it and about the exact form of the disease that you have—and what you can do about it. There are two excellent reasons to find a doctor and get a diagnosis. First, although hair loss is not usually a sign of a more serious disease, other causes of hair loss should be ruled out. Second, if you have a diagnosis of alopecia areata you can establish a relationship with a doctor who can help you, and you can begin to explore your options for treatment.

Hair Growth Phases for Normal Hair

The normal scalp contains an average of one hundred thousand hairs, of which between fifty and one hundred hairs are normally lost every day. Because there is constant regrowth of hair in the normal scalp, however, there is no overall net loss of hair. The hair follicles, as noted above, are the sacs containing the hairs. The normal follicle goes through a cycle of three phases: a growing phase, a transitional phase, and a resting phase.

At any given time about 90 percent of the hair follicles—and the hair—are in the growing phase (also called the *anagen* phase), which lasts between three and seven years. When the follicles reach the second phase (the transitional or *catagen* phase), the hair suddenly stops growing. This phase lasts approximately two to three weeks, and about 1 percent of the follicles are in this phase at any given time. This leaves between 8 and 10 percent of the follicles in the resting phase (also called the *telogen* phase), which lasts about three months. At the end of the telogen phase, the anagen growth (the new hair) pushes the telogen hair right out of the follicle and replaces it, and the cycle begins again. This replacement is part of the normal cycle of hair growth and accounts for the fifty to one hundred hairs that are lost daily from the scalp.

There are many reasons that some people lose more than the usual amount of hair: taking certain drugs, such as those used in treating cancer, can cause hair to fall out, for example. By far the most common cause of hair loss, however, is *androgenetic alopecia,* commonly known as male or female pattern baldness, which is completely different from alopecia areata. Androgenetic alopecia affects half of all men by age fifty and many women by the time they reach menopause. We all inherit genes that control what kind of hair we'll have, including the color, the texture (coarse, fine, curly, straight), and the density. Someone with androgenetic alopecia has inherited genes that express themselves as thinning hair or balding as the person ages.

In androgenetic alopecia, androgens, which are male hormones, cause the hair to become miniaturized as it grows through each cycle. The anagen phase becomes markedly reduced with each cycle, and so the hairs become smaller and smaller. In contrast, in alopecia areata the hairs are still very active underneath the scalp but can't get past the midphase of anagen growth. They prematurely go through catagen and telogen and reenter anagen, but the hair shaft does not have a chance to grow above the scalp, because the hair is "hibernating" underneath the scalp.

What Causes Alopecia Areata?

What causes alopecia areata? That's a good question, and one that many people are searching for an answer to.

In the past, alopecia areata research was not well funded, as this was not considered a serious health problem. But funding for alopecia areata research is catching up. Research efforts supported by private, corporate, and government funds are focused on trying to find the cause and the cure. Many published studies of the disease stem from a landmark event, the International Research Workshop on Alopecia Areata, which was held in October 1990. This workshop, which was cosponsored by the National Institute of Arthritis and Musculoskeletal and Skin Diseases (NIAMS) and the National Alopecia Areata Foundation (NAAF), brought dermatologists, immunologists, cell biologists, and biochemists together to summarize current research and define research goals. A repeat workshop in 1994 also stimulated more research in this area.

At this point, researchers have not yet pinpointed the cause of alopecia areata—or *causes,* because it's likely that alopecia is caused by a *combination* of genetic factors and external "triggers." For a long time, doctors thought that stress was the cause, but recent research has raised more questions than answers about the role of stress in alopecia areata. At present it appears that stress is much more likely to be a *result* of alopecia areata than a cause.

Doctors now think that alopecia areata is associated with a change in the immune system. This means that they consider alopecia areata to be an *autoimmune* disease. Medical researchers offer four pieces of evidence for this thinking. First, alopecia areata responds to a variety of treatments that alter the body's immune system. Whenever treatment designed to bring about a certain outcome works, then doctors can say with some assurance that the person did indeed have the disease or system malfunction that the treatment was designed to fix. If the symptoms of alopecia areata respond to treatment for a malfunctioning immune system—if the hair regrows—then it's fairly safe to say that the immune system is somehow involved in this disease. The immune system can be suppressed with drugs such as prednisone, a corticosteroid, and prednisone does in fact reverse hair loss in some people who have alopecia areata. But any drug that interferes with the functioning of the immune system over a prolonged period will lower the person's resistance to infection, creating a potentially very dangerous situation. There are, however, many unacceptable side effects of long-term use of prednisone, as we will see.

The second piece of evidence is that some people with alopecia areata have a higher than normal number of antibodies circulating in their blood. Antibodies are substances that the body produces in response to the action of a "foreign body." When the immune system goes on the defensive against a foreign invader in the body, such as a virus or material to which the person is allergic, it produces these antibodies to fight off the invader.

The third reason to believe that the immune system is involved is that cells interconnected with the immune system are found in the follicles of people with alopecia areata. When viewed under the microscope, the hair bulbs from a person with alopecia areata can be seen to be surrounded by inflammatory immune cells (called *T cells*), like a swarm of bees. *Langerhans' cells,* cells that present "foreign material" to the immune system, are usually absent in the deeper parts of the hair follicle, but they are present in people with alopecia areata. Also present in alopecia areata are *immune mediators,* biochemical signals involved in the immune system, which are not found in normal follicles.

There's one more measurable immune response: *HLA antigens.* When body tissue is under attack by the immune system, structures known as *histocompatibility antigens* (hence *HLA antigens,* which are measured with special diagnostic stains) are abnormally expressed, and this is exactly what happens with alopecia areata. With the remission of alopecia areata, Langerhans' cells, immune mediators, and HLA expression become normal.

Finally, people who have alopecia areata may be more likely to be diagnosed with another autoimmune disease, or to be related to someone with another autoimmune disease, than people who don't have alopecia areata. The incidence of autoimmune disease in people with alopecia areata is still very low, making this piece of evidence for involvement of the immune system in alopecia areata the weakest of the four. In a person with an autoimmune disease, the body's immune system produces antibodies that attack its own tissue. Rheumatoid arthritis is an autoimmune disease in which the body's immune system produces substances that erode the joints. Antibodies to thyroid, stomach, adrenal, and smooth muscle tissues appear to be two or three times more common in people with alopecia areata than in normal people.

If alopecia areata is an autoimmune process, then what's

the explanation for this autoimmune response, and what part of the follicle is being attacked by it? There are two possible explanations: either there is a change in the immune system or the hair follicle is abnormal. If the hair follicle is normal, then the problem would be found in the cells of the immune system, and the system would function as if it could not discriminate between what is self and nonself in the body—as a result, it would attack the follicles as if they were "not self." If the problem is in the follicle, then it may be a genetically determined, lifelong defect involving a component in or around the hair follicle that would lead the body to produce chemicals to maintain tissue damage.

Doctors and researchers don't yet know which of these two mechanisms is involved in alopecia areata, but for the reasons stated earlier, it's clear that the immune system is involved. Most researchers are leaning toward the second of these two mechanisms as the explanation. Their focus is on determining what part of the follicle is the target of the autoimmune response. Here there are four possibilities: the pigment cells (the melanocytes), the keratinocyte (another type of cell in the hair bulb), the cells of the dermal papilla (the cells in the portion of the dermis that is embraced by the hair bulb), or the cells that provide the blood circulation to the hair. In the past decade, many articles have been published implicating these various cells.

Some researchers have theorized that a microbial agent, such as a virus, could trigger an imbalance of immune responses and T cells in individuals who are genetically predisposed to develop alopecia areata. It is thought, for example, that some people who develop rheumatoid arthritis do so after having a bout with the flu; someone who was not genetically predisposed would recover from that same flu without developing rheumatoid arthritis, but for the predisposed person, the flu "activates" the disease process of rheumatoid arthritis. An association between alopecia areata and cytomegalovirus (CMV) recently has been postulated, but those data are still very inconclusive. In one preliminary study, the DNA of CMV was found to be increased in alopecia areata biopsies. Whether CMV is an innocent bystander or has portions of its structure similar to hair (molecular mimicry) still has to be worked out. There is no need to worry that alopecia areata is contagious or infectious, however.

Conditions That Sometimes Accompany Alopecia Areata

Most people with alopecia areata do not have any other disease, but a small proportion do, and these people have provided statistical information that has led doctors and researchers to identify probable links between alopecia areata and some other diseases, particularly those involving unusual immune system activity. The exact nature of the association between these diseases is not yet clear, but at this stage in the research it appears as if the association is correlational rather than causal: that is, we can only say that there is a *link* between alopecia and another disease; we can't say that one disease *causes* the other.

There's quite a bit of controversy swirling around

whether or not people with alopecia areata have a higher risk of having atopic conditions such as hay fever, asthma, and eczema. *Atopy* means having a genetic predisposition toward developing one of these allergic-type reactions. Atopy may be related to alopecia areata: it's possible that people with both alopecia areata and atopy are more likely to have a more severe or resistant form of alopecia areata.

There is also a correlation between alopecia areata and thyroid disease. Eight percent of people with alopecia areata have thyroid disease; this is higher than the incidence of thyroid disease in the general population, which is 2 percent. But even though there is a correlation between alopecia areata and thyroid disease, treating the thyroid disease does not remedy the alopecia areata.

Around 4 percent of people who have alopecia areata also experience a disease called *vitiligo,* or white spot, in contrast to a 1 percent incidence in the whole population. Someone with vitiligo will find that a small patch or larger area of skin loses its pigment and shows up paler than the surrounding skin. The immune system appears to be taking action against apparently normal skin cells. It's a disease that is difficult to treat, and it usually is permanent. Because vitiligo is more likely to develop on irritated skin, someone who has both alopecia areata and vitiligo may not be able to pursue certain treatment options for alopecia areata. Immunotherapy with diphenylcyclopropenone (diphencyprone), for example, irritates the skin and thus might make it more likely that vitiligo will appear in that area of the body.

Less than 10 percent of people with alopecia areata

have another autoimmune disease. As with all medical research, statistics may be significant or not. Several other diseases have been reported in case studies of people with alopecia areata; but when only one or two instances of a disease is reported, researchers can't conclude that there is therefore a link between alopecia areata and other diseases. Case studies have been reported of persons with alopecia areata also having or developing one or more of the following diseases: lupus erythematosus, rheumatoid arthritis, polymyalgia rheumatica, pemphigus foliaceous, hemolytic anemia, pernicious anemia, scleroderma, Addison's disease, thymoma, myasthenia gravis, ulcerative colitis, celiac disease, lichen sclerosus et atrophicus, hypogammaglobulinemia, and AIDS. These could just be coincidental diseases diagnosed in people with alopecia areata, or they could be in some way related to the immune alteration occurring in alopecia areata. More research is needed.

One encouraging piece of research is that a study of eight hundred people with alopecia areata showed a negative association with insulin-dependent diabetes mellitus, suggesting that alopecia areata may have a protective effect against this form of diabetes.

Alopecia Areata and Genetics

We know that genetic factors play a role in alopecia areata, because in people who have this condition, 20 percent can name one or more family member who has also been affected. A study from the Netherlands of 348 people with alopecia areata found that 7 percent of them had one parent affected, 3 percent had one sibling affected, and 2 percent had one child affected with a severe form of alopecia areata. In some cases, two or three—and even four—generations in one family have alopecia areata. In identical twins, sometimes both twins develop alopecia areata at the same time, sometimes in the same part of the scalp. All of this provides evidence to support a belief that there's a genetic factor that plays a role in determining who gets alopecia areata.

Many dermatologists believe that only a certain proportion of the population has the genetic makeup that makes them susceptible to, or able to develop, alopecia areata, and that in these persons exposure to various immune trigger factors may lead them to develop alopecia areata. Certain genetic groups with a particular type of HLA gene (these genes are found on chromosome 6) appear to have a higher chance of having severe disease. Testing for this HLA gene (called gene "typing") is not yet a practical laboratory test for people with alopecia areata, but it is an experimental tool that helps research scientists to understand the genetic makeup of the condition.

Alopecia Areata of the Nails

If fingernail and toenail changes occur in people with alopecia, those people are said to have *alopecia areata of the nails*. Depending on which report you read, between 2 and 50 percent of people with alopecia areata have nail changes; the wide variation in these reports probably depends on how much time and attention is spent looking for the nail changes. Those with more widespread hair loss have a greater chance of having nail changes, so children, who frequently have more severe alopecia, have a higher risk of nail distortion. These changes may persist after the hair has regrown, and they may occur before or at the same time as the hair loss.

The most common nail change that may occur with alopecia is an almost invisible pitting—as if a pin has made tiny dents in the nail. Less common changes are ridging (from top to bottom of nail), rough or sandpaper nails (trachyonychia), or white or red spots at the base of the nail. In rare cases, the nail plate may separate from the nail bed (onycholysis), or in very rare cases the nail may be completely lost (onychomadesis). Spoon-shaped nails have also been reported.

Diagnosing Alopecia Areata

People with alopecia areata almost always seek help from a doctor when they begin to notice an unusual pattern of hair loss or a large amount of hair loss. In addition to the three patterns noted above, there are other variations in the way alopecia areata affects people. Some people lose substantial amounts of hair very quickly—within a few weeks. This is called the *acute* phase of alopecia areata. People with *subacute* alopecia areata have slow hair loss, occurring over many months. In either of these cases the hair may regrow spontaneously, and the problem is resolved. But for some people the loss is *chronic*, meaning that it lasts for many months, years, or decades. The chronic forms of alopecia areata can be divided into two subtypes: stable forms with no change for years, or regrowth and hair loss occurring simultaneously or at different times on different areas of the scalp and body.

Hairless areas of skin on the scalp caused by alopecia areata usually look just like normal skin. In Caucasians, sometimes the color is closer to ivory, or it is peach colored or (rarely) red. The subtle changes are not usually apparent on black skin. A soft swelling of the scalp can sometimes be felt in these areas. Most people don't notice any sensation associated with hair loss, but some feel an itch, tingling, or slight local pain shortly before the hair begins to fall out or on the area where the hair has fallen out.

The pattern of hair loss on the scalp can take many different shapes. The most common is a well-defined circular patch (though not necessarily perfectly circular). The bare patches are not scarred, and the pores from which the hair usually emerges can be easily seen. There are other, less common, patterns of alopecia areata, such as a netlike arrangement, in which irregular areas without hair are interspersed with areas of hair on the scalp. Or the disease may show up as diffuse but incomplete hair loss over the entire scalp. This pattern looks like hair that is simply thinning, without any bald patches. Another form of the disease is known as *ophiasis,* which means a snake or band of hair loss around the periphery or margins of the scalp. People with this pattern of hair loss may develop more severe hair loss, and fingernails and toenails may be affected.

When someone sees a doctor because of any of these patterns of hair loss, the doctor usually can easily make a diagnosis. Alopecia areata is characterized by the well-defined round patches of hair loss. Within those patches, the doctor may see "exclamation point" hairs—broken-off short hairs that taper (get narrower) toward the scalp. Making a diagnosis of alopecia areata is more difficult in someone with diffuse hair loss or with different kinds of hair loss occurring simultaneously. In this case, the doctor may want to take a biopsy of the scalp, to determine the exact diagnosis.

To take a biopsy, the doctor will remove a piece of skin from the scalp the size and shape of a pencil eraser, usually using a four-millimeter punch biopsy. It is minimally painful and sounds worse than it is. The punch biopsy is a cookie-cutter–like instrument that cuts through the skin down to the fat. Before taking the biopsy, the doctor will inject anesthetic into the skin; the injection usually burns like a bee sting for a brief period, but it's worth it, since it also makes the biopsy almost painless. After the piece of skin is taken, the small hole is sewn up with a few stitches. The specimen of skin is sent to a pathologist who will use a microscope to examine the hair follicles from skin surface to hair root, looking for unusual immune cell activity to indicate a diagnosis of alopecia areata, and for changes characteristic of other hair loss problems.

What Is the Prognosis?

One of the most difficult aspects of alopecia areata, both for the doctor and for the person who has it, is its uncertain and capricious course. For most people, small amounts of hair fall out, then regrow within months. But it's difficult to predict, for any one individual, what the course and duration of the disease will be. It may be acute and short-lived, with regrowth in some sites and loss in others. Much less commonly, it may be fulminant—developing very swiftly, with progression from a few patches to total or universal hair loss in a matter of days or weeks.

There's a possibility of spontaneous hair regrowth for years after alopecia areata first develops, even for people who lose all of their hair. But there's no telling when or how much regrowth might occur, or how long the new hair will last, for any given individual. The following examples demonstrate the apparently random course and extent of this frustrating disease.

A woman in her forties lost approximately 80 percent of her hair when she moved to another country with her husband, but all her hair grew back within six months. Now in her sixties, this woman has never had a recurrence of alopecia areata.

A boy six years of age developed one patch of alopecia areata, and then hair regrew on that spot. Throughout his school days he had periods of full hair and periods when he had one or more small bald patches, often on different areas of his scalp. He received steroid injections in the bald patches during his teenage years, and hair regrew. After three years of having a full head of hair, suddenly half his hair fell out. Since then, he has had extensive bald areas that rove around his scalp, changing shape as new hairs regrow and other hairs fall out.

A woman in her twenties developed two bald patches that regrew when treated with steroid injections. A few months later, about 25 percent of her scalp hair fell out, and the injections did not stimulate regrowth. Four years later, all her body and scalp hair fell out, and she was diagnosed with alopecia universalis. Treatment with minoxidil (Rogaine) and then with diphenylcyclopropenone brought a few hairs back, but not enough to be cosmetically acceptable. She stopped the treatments. After three years, hair began to regrow on her arms; the following year her eyebrows and eyelashes grew back, and in the last three years she has begun to regrow hair on her scalp and pubic area.

Once someone has developed alopecia areata, there are three possible outcomes: spontaneous remission, continual disease, or flare-up (or recurrence) of disease after a period of remission. *Remission* is the term used to describe a disease when it subsides into an inactive state which may last an undetermined length of time. Someone who has had one occurrence of alopecia areata may be free of it for the rest of his or her life, or may have recurrences of hair loss in the same body area or in other body areas at various times throughout his or her life.

Why alopecia areata progresses and regresses is not yet known. Another problem is that, while certain observations may be made based on what doctors know about what *usually* happens when someone has a certain pattern and form of hair loss, unusual events do occur, making any prediction susceptible to error. Considering how uncertain the prognosis is, the best advice we can give is, again, to seek a diagnosis, and then receive treatment that is appropriate for the particular pattern and form of the disease that you have.

Treating Alopecia Areata

There is no cure for alopecia areata yet, but there are effective treatments. Most people regrow hair at some point, either through treatment or through spontaneous remission. The goal of research in the treatment of alopecia areata is to determine the specific antigen that is responsible for the disease (an antigen is a protein or carbohydrate substance that can stimulate an immune response). When that antigen is discovered, treatment can become specifically targeted to suppressing it; in the meantime, treatment is a bit like hitting a nail with a sledgehammer, because *nonspecific* immunological therapies must be used. These treatments often work, but some of them affect the whole body, not just the hair, and therefore they can cause a variety of side effects. When researchers manage to identify the specific immunological antigen or mediator that needs to be blocked, it will revolutionize therapy: doctors will be able to provide specific treatment directed at the exact cause of the disease.

On the other hand, there have been many promising developments in the treatment of alopecia areata in the last decade, especially in the treatment of chronic severe alopecia areata, which was considered untreatable by most dermatologists only fifteen years ago. Steroids were the only form of treatment available in the 1970s, but treatments such as topical and systemic immunotherapy, minoxidil, anthralin, and photochemotherapy have since been added to the medical armamentarium.

Some people find that as their hair is regrowing, new

patches of hair loss may appear. The treatments for this disease may stimulate hair growth without controlling or halting the disease process, and discontinuing the treatment often means losing the new hair growth. On the other hand, if the disease goes completely into remission, the treatment can be discontinued.

As is true of treatments for many other medical conditions, the treatment and resulting hair growth in alopecia areata should be closely monitored by a doctor. Your doctor is the best person to determine when treatment should be started and stopped, and you should visit him or her regularly for an examination and consultation. You can also help your doctor—and yourself—by keeping a record of treatments and their effectiveness as well as keeping track of your hair loss and growth.

What are the factors taken into consideration when determining what treatment is best for any one individual? The extent of hair loss is one of the most important factors; others are the person's age, general health, psychological state, occupation, and personal feelings about the hair loss, which will affect his or her motivation for sticking with a treatment that may or may not succeed. For the most successful outcome, the individual and his or her family doctor or dermatologist should take all of these factors into account when deciding about treatment.

The treatment of alopecia areata has changed dramatically in the past decade. There are new options that were not available only a short time ago, and researchers are pursuing more new treatments. Your family doctor or dermatologist will probably describe the treatment options that are right for you, and tell you about their potential success and side effects. If this doesn't happen, be sure to ask, and if you're not satisfied, consider getting a second opinion. You will want to gather all the information you can before making a decision about your treatment.

Developing a Treatment Plan

The patient is always given the option of having no treatment, since there is a 60 percent chance of spontaneous resolution within two years. In fact, a controlled study of 119 patients with alopecia areata affecting less than 40 percent of their scalp showed that using a placebo was just as effective as topical immunotherapy with squaric acid dibutylester or diphenylcyclopropenone or topical 1 percent minoxidil.

It's very important to remember that spontaneous remission occurs in many people with less severe alopecia areata when interpreting the results of *uncontrolled* studies of various therapies for alopecia areata. Uncontrolled studies lack a standard for comparison, such as a similar group of patients with alopecia areata who are observed over time without treatment or, in a person with alopecia totalis, an "untreated half" of the scalp. Without such controls, it is never clear whether the treated patients responded to the treatment or just had spontaneous hair regrowth. The rate of spontaneous regrowth must also be considered when treating people with less severe alopecia areata; however, we believe that intralesional corticosteroid therapy does accelerate resolution of the condition if the long-term prognosis is favorable.

There are many different approaches to treating alopecia areata, determined in part by where (in what country, and in what part of that country) a physician has been educated and trained as well as where he or she is currently practicing. A physician in private practice will be guided by the results of studies as reported in the medical literature and also by his or her own experience about what has been successful. Physicians who are in a group practice or who practice in a hospital or clinic setting may follow a protocol for treatment that has been established by the members of the group or clinic. In this book we are describing the treatment protocol in use at the University of British Columbia Hair Clinic, but we can say with assurance that other approaches to treatment are used, and that they are effective.

At the UBC Hair Clinic, treatment decisions are based on what the clinic staff consider to be the two most important factors: (1) extent of the hair loss and (2) age. Extent is divided into two categories: (1) more than 50 percent scalp hair loss and (2) less than 50 percent scalp hair loss. Age is also divided into two categories, adults and children (under twelve years of age).

Adults with Less Than 50 Percent Scalp Hair Loss

For adults with less than 50 percent scalp hair loss, treatment options include the following, in order of preference:

1. Intralesional corticosteroids: injecting small amounts of corticosteroids into the affected scalp areas as well as the eyebrow area for those who have lost eyebrows
2. Minoxidil solution (Rogaine at its medical strength) alone

3. Combination therapy
  a. Minoxidil solution and corticosteroid cream
  b. Minoxidil solution and anthralin
4. Topical immunotherapy

Now let's look more closely at each of these four treatment options.

1. **Intralesional corticosteroids.** For alopecia areata, intralesional corticosteroid injections (injections of corticosteroids) remain the treatment of choice when less than 50 percent of the scalp is involved. Most dermatologists prefer to use triamcinolone acetonide (Kenalog), a corticosteroid that can be injected directly into the skin. The concentrations used in different treatment centers varies, from 2.5 mg/ml to 10 mg/ml. The higher the concentration the greater the chance of denting of the scalp. At the UBC Hair Clinic, we prefer a concentration of 5 mg/ml, and we recommend that a maximum total of 2 ml be given, with multiple injections of 0.1 ml each, approximately 1 centimeter apart, with a half-inch-long 30–gauge needle.

The treatments are repeated every four to six weeks and, because they are well tolerated by adults, they can be repeated indefinitely. The success rate with scalp injections in selected patients is approximately 70 percent. In the 30 percent in whom there are no results after the second set of injections, our next choice of treatment is topical minoxidil. For eyebrows, a 2.5 mg/ml concentration of triamcinolone acetonide is used. Half a milliliter is injected into each eyebrow, with five injections of 0.1 ml each. Eyebrow treatments are done monthly.

2. **Minoxidil.** Minoxidil was originally used, and con-

tinues to be used, to reduce high blood pressure. It is also used topically (applied on the skin) for androgenetic alopecia (male or female pattern baldness). It has also been used with some success in treating alopecia areata, although success varies with the extent of alopecia and the concentration of the minoxidil solution used. Higher dosage appears to increase the response rate. There is some evidence from controlled studies to suggest that results that are acceptable to the patient can be expected in approximately 14 percent of cases with extensive alopecia areata (75–90 percent hair loss) and in approximately 48 percent of cases with patchy alopecia (less than 75 percent hair loss).

The 2 percent formula of minoxidil that currently is widely available is most likely to elicit cosmetically acceptable regrowth in people with patchy alopecia. An acceptable response should not be expected if the current episode of alopecia areata has lasted longer than ten years or if hair loss is total (100 percent). The average time to respond with initial growth of terminal (coarse, thickened) hairs is three months, with an average of 62 weeks' constant use required for full regrowth.

Minoxidil is applied every twelve hours. At the University of British Columbia, the 5 percent minoxidil solution is used almost exclusively, because the literature reports significantly better results with this higher concentration. If there are no results after twelve weeks of minoxidil, the next step is combination therapy.

Minoxidil may cost up to thirty dollars per month (a 60 cc bottle usually lasts one month) for the generic 2 percent or 5 percent solution. The generic solution is not available in the United States yet, but it is available in Canada and most countries in Europe, except Germany. Rogaine (2 percent minoxidil solution, manufactured by the Pharmacia & Upjohn Company in Kalamazoo, Michigan) is the only minoxidil that is available in the United States. As of April 15, 1996, it has been approved for over-the-counter use (without perscription).

Most insurance companies will not reimburse for minoxidil, because it is not an FDA-approved therapy for alopecia areata, meaning that the manufacturer of the product has not demonstrated to the FDA that it is an effective treatment. However, if your doctor fills out certain forms (referred to in the appendix), then the purchase of minoxidil may be reimbursed.

3. Combination therapy. Minoxidil can be used in combination with a topically applied corticosteroid cream, in which case the cream may increase the penetration of the minoxidil solution by covering it. At the UBC Hair Clinic, patients are told to apply betamethasone dipropionate cream twice daily, thirty minutes after each use of 5 percent minoxidil solution. Some good results have been found with combination therapy, sometimes better than with monotherapy (using either of these two agents alone), indicating that the two agents may act synergistically. In some studies, success rates as high as 50 percent have been reported; at the UBC Hair Clinic, however, the success rate with a combination of betamethasone dipropionate cream and minoxidil solution has only been 25 percent. (We should note that this is an uncontrolled study.)

If this combination does not work after twelve weeks, at the UBC Hair Clinic the next step is a combination of 1 percent anthralin cream applied for one hour, then thoroughly washed off, and 5 percent minoxidil applied twice a day. Anthralin cream is a chemical used to treat psoriasis. It may act as an immunomodulator (modulating the immune system). Studies have shown a synergistic effect with this combination, with new hair growth appearing within three months, while the average length of time for cosmetic hair growth response was twenty-three weeks. At the UBC Hair Clinic the reported good success of the anthralin-minoxidil combination has eluded most of our patients, but since success has been reported elsewhere, we continue to prescribe this regimen. If after twelve weeks there is no regrowth, topical immunotherapy is used. The side effects of anthralin are irritation and brown staining of the skin and staining of clothes and bedsheets.

4. **Topical immunotherapy.** Some other chemicals have stimulated hair growth in some people. These chemicals—diphenylcyclopropenone, dinitrochlorobenzene, and squaric acid dibutylester—affect the immune system in a way that's similar to the way poison ivy affects the immune system. *Topical immunotherapy,* as this treatment is called, is not easy to obtain in the United States and usually must be performed under strict medical supervision. Diphenylcyclopropenone may soon become more easily available in the United States, however. For a complete description of this treatment, see below.

Adults with More Than 50 Percent Scalp Hair Loss

At the UBC Hair Clinic, for adults with more than 50 percent scalp hair loss, the following treatment options are used (in order of preference):

1. Topical immunotherapy
2. Topical immunotherapy—combined with intralesional corticosteroids to areas not responding to topical immunotherapy alone
3. Combination therapy—minoxidil solution and corticosteroid cream or minoxidil solution and anthralin
4. PUVA
5. Systemic corticosteroids

1. **Topical immunotherapy.** For adults with more than 50 percent hair loss, topical immunotherapy with diphenylcyclopropenone is the treatment of choice at the UBC Hair Clinic as well as at many European university dermatology centers. Topical immunotherapy uses an *immunogen,* a substance similar to an antigen, which is capable of producing a response from the immune system. Topical immunotherapy is the most effective treatment with the best safety profile in the treatment of chronic severe alopecia areata. Systemic steroids such as prednisone may be the most effective treatment, but the level of safety with systemic steroids is unacceptable to most dermatologists. Three contact sensitizers have been used extensively: diphenylcyclopropenone (DPCP), dinitrochlorobenzene (DNCB), and squaric acid dibutylester (SADBE). At the University of British Columbia, DPCP is used because it is the least expensive and the most stable.

Just how topical immunotherapy works in the treatment of alopecia areata is unclear. A number of theories have been proposed. It may be that the immunogen (the chemical substance that produces the immunity) attracts a new population of T cells into the treated area of the scalp, helping to clear away the hair follicle antigen that is being attacked in alopecia areata. An alternative explanation involves the concept of "antigenic competition." In the presence of the chemically introduced immunogen, it may be that nonspecific T cells are generated in the area which inhibit the autoimmune reaction to the hair-associated antigen, allowing hair to regrow.

By some as yet not completely understood mechanism, then, immunogens seem to interfere with the process that is causing alopecia areata by causing an allergic reaction to occur. Along with hair growth, this allergic reaction causes a dermatitis—redness and itching of the scalp. If we knew exactly which component of the multifaceted allergic reaction suppressed alopecia areata, it might be possible to understand what exactly is going on with alopecia areata.

In dermatology, DPCP has been used not only in the treatment of alopecia areata, but also as an immunomodulator in the treatment of melanoma and warts. Its effectiveness with alopecia areata varies from study to study. The largest study of patients with severe alopecia areata—the majority with almost total, totalis, or universalis type—was conducted by Pieter van der Steen and Associates in 139 patients and reported a response rate of 50.4 percent with cosmetically acceptable results.

In this study, the following three factors had a negative influence on the success of the treatment. First was the extent of hair loss. Scalp involvement of 40–90 percent had a response rate of approximately 75 percent, but for more extensive hair loss, the response rate was 40 percent. The second factor was the duration of alopecia areata before treatment. Response rate was reduced in cases of longer duration. Finally, if the patient had nail changes, treatment was not as successful.

Factors such as age of onset, sex, presence of atopic features, and extent of variation in the range of DPCP concentrations during treatment did not influence the prognosis significantly. Thirty of 139 patients had the disease return to one side of their head during treatment of the entire scalp and were resistant to further therapy. In eight of 139 patients a "tolerance" phenomenon was observed, in which, in order to continue to grow hair, the patients needed a continuous increase in DPCP concentration until a concentration of 2 percent was reached without producing an adequate dermatitis, resulting in the loss of all regrown hair.

In 1988, studies done by Susan MacDonald-Hull showed hair growth in fourteen of twenty-eight patients (a 50 percent success rate on the treated side of the scalp), with eight of twenty-eight (29 percent) showing a cosmetically acceptable result. In a 1989 study of posttherapy relapse rate within six months after treatment, MacDonald-Hull found that seven of nineteen (37 percent) showed no hair loss after treatment had been stopped for six months. In 68 percent, the appearance of the scalp six months later was cosmetically acceptable, although 53 percent developed patchy alopecia and 10 percent lost all hair that had regrown. In 1991, Macdonald-Hull reported additional results with DPCP used on a larger number of people, in which she found that forty-nine of seventy-eight patients (62 percent) showed regrowth of hair. Twenty-five of the seventy-eight (32 percent) showed complete regrowth of hair. This researcher is convinced that eliciting an allergic reaction is an integral part of successful treatment resulting in hair growth.

The first North American study of DPCP, conducted by Jerry Shapiro with others, reported a success rate of fourteen of forty patients (35 percent) in severe alopecia areata (more than 50 percent scalp hair loss). All fourteen of these patients abandoned their wigs over an eight- to ten-month period. Those who had the disease less than one year and who did not have alopecia universalis tended to do better. Since 1989, Shapiro has treated over 120 patients with similar results.

DPCP is used at the UBC Hair Clinic as follows. It is applied initially as a 2 percent solution onto a four centimeter by four centimeter area on one side of the scalp. Individuals return weekly. After one week, if no reaction or only a mild reaction is observed, a 0.0001 percent solution is applied to only half of the scalp. If there is a marked reaction, no solution is applied until the following week. The DPCP is left on the scalp for forty-eight hours and then washed off. The patient is advised to protect the scalp from light for at least thirty-six hours but preferably for a full forty-eight hours because DPCP is degraded when exposed to light.

The following week, DPCP is reapplied to the same half of the scalp. The aim is to maintain erythema (redness) and pruritus (itching) on the treated side for twenty-four to thirty-six hours after application. The concentration is adjusted individually depending on the severity of the previous reaction. Concentrations will vary (0.0001 percent, 0.001 percent, 0.01 percent, 0.05 percent, 0.1 percent, 0.5 percent, 1.0 percent, 2.0 percent). Once hair growth has been established on one side of the scalp, the other side is treated. The patient returns weekly. Once full regrowth is achieved, treatment can be given less frequently.

Side effects of topical immunotherapy include eczema, autoeczematization, severe blistering, and lymphadenopathy (swollen nodes) in the neck and behind the ears. (Eczema is redness of the skin with tiny, medium-sized, or large water blisters; autoeczematization is spreading eczema affecting larger areas of the body other than the scalp.) Contact urticaria (wheals or hives), vitiligo, decreased pigment or increased pigment, and other, less common, reactions have also been reported.

Before beginning this treatment, people should become thoroughly informed about its experimental nature, the lack of sufficient information about potentially toxic effects of the treatment, the chances for hair regrowth, the possible side effects, and the possible failure to respond. People must be warned that the induction of an allergic contact dermatitis is a desired outcome of the treatment, and one that is necessary to achieve a good result. A local ethics committee (for example, a hospital investigation review board) should be asked for consent. If the treating physician has obtained approval from a local ethics committee, the patient will usually be asked to sign a consent form that describes the risks and benefits of the treatment.

2. **Topical immunotherapy with corticosteroid injections.** When topical immunotherapy is working in only parts of the scalp, injections of corticosteroids may be given to the areas of the scalp that are not responding. If, after twenty-four weeks, topical immunotherapy is unsuccessful, another treatment protocol will be started.

3. **Combination therapy** (combining topical minoxidil and either topical corticosteroid or anthralin) has been discussed earlier in this chapter.

4. PUVA. PUVA is an acronym representing a form of phototherapy. The *P* denotes *psoralen,* a drug that causes extreme sensitivity to intense sun exposure. The *UVA* refers to *ultraviolet A* radiation, a portion of the sun's spectrum that causes suntanning. PUVA therapy is commonly used to treat severe psoriasis, and some physicians use it to treat severe alopecia areata. At the UBC Hair Clinic, the rate of success is only about 10 percent, but other centers have reported success rates as high as 50 percent. The way this treatment works on alopecia areata is that PUVA may have an effect on the immune system.

For treatment, the drug psoralen is administered either topically (0.1 percent 8-MOP cream or 1 percent 8-MOP lotion) or orally (0.6 mg/kg 8-MOP). One or two hours later, the patient receives irradiation with UVA by standing in a sun lamp booth (8-MOP, or 8-methoxy-psoralen, is a chemical that makes the skin more sensitive to the long wavelengths of the ultraviolet light spectrum). Treatments are administered two to three times a week, with gradual increase in UVA dosage.

Side effects that may occur within days of treatment include sunburn and blistering of the skin, and conjunctivitis of the eyes, if proper eye protection is not used. Long-term side effects usually occur after more than a year of treatment and include premature aging of the skin, nonmelanoma skin cancers, and ocular cataracts, if proper eye protection is not used. The effectiveness of local PUVA using topical psoralen application, as well as systemic PUVA using oral ingestion of psoralen, in treating alopecia areata is controversial. Many physicians who do use PUVA believe that local treatment with topical psoralen is not as effective as systemic treatment with oral psoralen, which, in theory, has a much greater effect on the abnormal immune response. One major problem with PUVA is that most patients who do respond after several months of treatment three times every week have their hair fall out when they stop therapy, and so they must continue active therapy to maintain their hair growth.

5. **Systemic corticosteroids.** Short-term therapy (lasting a few weeks to several weeks) with systemic corticosteroids (steroids taken by mouth) frequently causes temporary hair regrowth. Unfortunately, hair shedding is usually seen when the systemic treatment is discontinued. For this reason, a second form of therapy is almost always used in conjunction with short-term systemic corticosteroid therapy, in hopes that the second therapy will maintain the effect seen with corticosteriods once the systemic corticosteroids are discontinued.

Long-term corticosteroid treatment is not used because of the demonstrated side effects and the fact that the drug does not alter the long-term prognosis. In children, one significant—and unacceptable—side effect of long-term use of systemic steroids is stunted growth. Other potential side effects that make this an inappropriate long-term therapy for both children and adults are weight gain, high blood pressure, diabetes, ulcer disease, osteoporosis (thinning of the bones), and ocular cataracts and glaucoma. At the UBC Hair Clinic, systemic steroids are used only in exceptional cases. In fact, systemic prednisone has been used in only two cases in the last ten years.

Children Younger Than Age Twelve

For children younger than twelve years of age with alopecia areata, the treatments used at the UBC Hair Clinic are:

1. Minoxidil
2. Minoxidil with topical corticosteroid
3. Minoxidil with anthralin

Minoxidil 5 percent solution is the first therapy choice for children (again, the cutoff for children is age twelve), followed by combination therapy of minoxidil and either betamethasone dipropionate cream or anthralin.

Many dermatologists are reluctant to use topical immunotherapy with chemicals such as DPCP on children, because it is still an experimental therapy. Many are also reluctant to inject cortisone into children, because of the pain of the injections. And, because of the side effects described above, long-term systemic steroid therapy is not an option: systemic steroids must never be used in children for the treatment of alopecia areata.

Although corticosteroids used topically or intralesionally are much safer, they may cause undesirable side effects on the areas where they are applied, such as thinning of the skin, stretch marks, dilated blood vessels, and folliculitis. They may (rarely) even cause the effects seen with systemic corticosteroids. For these reasons, physician monitoring is essential when continuous therapy is used, in children and in adults.

Need for Treatment, Need for Hope

Alopecia areata is a disease for which orthodox medicine has not discovered a cure—yet. Orthodox treatments range from the mostly successful and safe to the sometimes successful and mostly safe, through treatments that require a careful balancing of the benefits of regrowing hair with the documented medical side effects. Some treatments require the use of caution and judgment in deciding when and for how long to utilize them. It's not the most hopeful of situations, and yet hope is essential to maintain motivation to cope well.

In addition, there is still much to be learned about the normal physiology of hair as well as the abnormal, or "pathophysiology," of alopecia areata. The more studies are done, the more clearly we see the limits of our knowledge about all aspects of body and image. But a situation that blends ignorance, uncertainty, and the need for hope is ripe ground for unproven remedies.

Bombarded with Advice

When a person develops alopecia areata, he or she may be bombarded with advice. Older family members may offer up folk remedies, such as brushing the remaining hair (or scalp) one hundred times a day; work colleagues may suggest paying a visit to a pricey beauty salon advertising scalp massages to "strengthen" hair; friends may advise taking specific vitamins or supplements. Advertisements from hair replacement clinics, backed with glowing testimonials, appear in many newspapers and magazines. The person with alopecia areata may even be told that orthodox doctors are so useless, that those in the medical establishment should be avoided in favor of practitioners of "alternative" therapies, such as homeopathy or colonic irrigation. All of this advice can be totally bewildering.

Quacks and Miracle Cures

One of the few entertaining things about having alopecia areata is finding out just what people have been recommending down through the centuries to hold onto this stuff on our scalps—or get it to grow back. Some of the remedies are thousands of years old, showing that hair loss—whatever the cause—has been a source of anxiety for people as long as we have records. The recipes make us glad to be alive these days, rather than in simpler but messier olden times.

To give readers a sense of the variety of ancient remedies used to treat hair loss, Albert Kligman and Beth Freeman listed the following in an article in the journal

Clinics in Dermatology (vol. 6, no. 4, 1988): spider webs; dog urine; oil of wormwood; bear grease and laudanum; German army horse saliva; equal parts of Abyssinian greyhound's heel, date blossoms, and ass's hoof—boiled in oil; equal parts of fat of a lion, a hippopotamus, a crocodile, a goose, a snake, and an ibex. All of these remedies, we hope, were applied topically rather than ingested. Kligman and Freeman also cited intriguing national variations in approaches to treatment: fresh bovine heart and lecithins in Germany; vitamins in Japan; horseradish, mustard oil, citrus peel, and egg yolk in Hungary; and acupuncture in the former Soviet Union. Richard Sandomir, in his book *Bald like Me,* includes his own compendium of strange cures, including dew from the traditional healing plant St. John's wort, and Cleopatra's remedy—burned domestic mice, horse teeth, bear grease, and deer marrow. Sandomir points out that this latter potion doesn't seem to have worked for Cleopatra's love, Julius Caesar, who was anxious about his baldness for most of his life.

Trichoquackery

Here's a word that every person with alopecia needs to learn: *trichoquackery.* You won't find it in the dictionary, but it's been coined, through necessity, to cover nonorthodox "remedies" for hair loss. The root word, *tricho* (Greek for hair), is found in the word *trichology,* meaning the study of hair. The *quackery* in *trichoquackery* comes from the great traditions of quacks who for so long have peddled snake oil and other "cures" for hair loss. In other words, trichoquackery describes the multitude of remedies that haven't been proven to work.

Nonorthodox approaches come in many different forms: recipes (or special shampoos), either manufactured or self-mixed, to rub onto the scalp; practices such as stimulating the scalp (by massage or by tapping with a hairbrush); and various other approaches, ranging from homeopathy to acupuncture to relaxation techniques to psychotherapy to vitamin therapy to having one's mercury fillings replaced in case this has caused the immune system to malfunction.

Alternative Medicine

Many alternative therapies do not treat symptoms or disease. For them, the overriding concern is the whole person. Their philosophy is that "the person who has the disease is more important than the disease that has the person"—so in the hands of these practitioners you will be treated as a whole, and the alopecia will be seen as a sign of some kind of imbalance. All parts of the person—body, mind, and emotions—will be taken into consideration.

Some of these alternative therapies are making a comeback as more and more people are turning to herbs and other "natural" drugs. Like other alternative therapies, some of these are benign, some can be harmful, and some may have some good effects, if not on hair loss, then on stress or other conditions. Some medical doctors are hopeful about the promise of such treatments, but some are concerned that they will do more harm than good.

Naturopathy. A naturopath is a person, sometimes a medical doctor, who advises on "lifestyle" changes, such as diet (in detail), sleep problems, anxiety, unproductive behavior patterns, and exercise. The idea is that when you find the lifestyle that is right for you—and who these days can say they have a fulfilled and not overly stressful life?—symptoms of imbalance should disappear. This is generally a healthy thing to do, unlikely to cause harm, and may well improve your energy and emotional life.

Homeopathy. Homeopathy is a system of therapeutics founded in the nineteenth century as a way of "treating like with like"—that is, if you show symptoms of something, you will be treated with something that would produce the same effect, but the substance (in the form of a powder or pill) is given in tiny amounts in an attempt to stimulate the body's own defenses to work out the health problem. It's similar to the concept of vaccination. Conventional immunotherapy is similar to homeopathy but does not involve the use of "natural" products.

As in naturopathic medicine, the homeopathic healer may or may not be a medical doctor, and he or she treats the whole person, not the symptom. It is unlikely that ten people with alopecia areata would be treated with the same remedy; rather, each would have his or her own personal remedy that takes the many other aspects of him or her—and not just hair loss—into consideration. Homeopathy is believed to be safe because the amounts given as treatment are so diluted that, as yet, there is *no scientific* explanation as to how they could have any effect at all.

Hair Cosmetics. While anything labeled as a guaranteed cure for hair loss should be approached in a spirit of skepticism, some hair stylists are adept at minimizing thinning or patchy alopecia areata by using mousses, vitamin-enriched hair thickeners, scalp dyes, and other products or practices. Alopecia-masking lotions for bald areas can be used to camouflage alopecia areata. Clever haircuts or permanent waves, or even changing the color of the hair so that the scalp is less noticeable, sometimes minimize a problem.

What to Do?

In this atmosphere of ignorance, uncertainty, claim and counterclaim, and side effects, untested hair loss remedies are still big business. People have different attitudes toward alternative treatments. For some, whatever remedy they try is a positive thing to do as long as it helps them to cope and tilts the balance toward hope rather than despair. Whatever the treatment, however age-hallowed and highly recommended, the fact remains that in scientific terms, *none of the nonmedical remedies have been proven to grow hair.* If any of them had, you can be sure that a large pharmaceutical company would have tested it themselves and told the world about it. After all, if there were a remedy that regrew hair, it would make those involved with its discovery and manufacture very wealthy indeed.

The main thing to remember is that alopecia areata is a disease, and, as such, it is a totally different kind of hair loss from pattern baldness or stress-induced thinning. The view under the microscope makes this quite clear. If a product has efficacy for male pattern baldness, it may not work for people with alopecia areata, so they need to appraise carefully any claims that are made for unproven remedies.

When it comes to deciding whether to spend time, money, and emotional energy on any alternative to orthodox medicine, it's good to remember that, generally speaking, the less someone promises, the more trustworthy he or she is. Also, there is often a difference between what is implied and what is actually stated. Photos can be faked. Statistics can mean anything. Claims about a product or practice such as "Regrows hair" or "Grows new hair" may actually mean something like "One person (who may not have had alopecia areata) out of six hundred got a lot of vellus hair ('peach fuzz') on his scalp for a few days. It only cost him sixty hours annually and $5,000."

The most important thing about trying unproven treatments is to be very, very careful. Doctors often warn patients against unproven treatments because they have seen people over the years spend huge amounts of money on unregulated and vaguely defined pots of gunk to put on their scalp or, an even more expensive option, gunk that can be applied only through certain technologies (such as heat or manual massage) that require repeated visits to salons and the repeated expense of having someone apply the gunk.

All medical doctors will tell you before treatment begins that there are no guarantees in the treatment of alopecia areata. Anyone who "guarantees" results ought to be willing to refund your money if the results are not satisfactory according to some *agreed upon* definition of *satisfactory.*

Hairpieces and Headcovers

Wig, "hair," toupee, rug—whatever you call it, a hairpiece can help you feel better about yourself. If you're embarrassed or feel unattractive because you have lost your hair, wearing a wig can help. It will improve your appearance and boost your confidence and self-esteem. And, just as a roof protects the contents of your house, a wig can shelter you from cold, sun, rain—and, perhaps most important, from stares. A wig protects your head and your feelings. Just like glasses or contact lenses, a wig helps you to function better (that's why a wig is sometimes called a *cranial prosthesis*), and it can be as essential to your quality of life as corrective lenses. Wearing a wig or toupee marks a significant turning point in your life.

In eighteenth-century Europe, wigs were *the* fashion accessory. People with thick hair shaved their heads so they could wear a wig, preferably as high on the forehead as possible. Similarly, in the entertainment industry today, wigs and "pieces," weaves and extensions, are commonly used by both men and women. Think about it—not all those Hollywood stars were born with big, glamorous hair. What this all adds up to is a long tradition of wig wearing to enhance appearance. When you wear a wig, you can consider yourself part of an elite set.

If you are a woman, your hairpiece doesn't have to limit

your image: you can experiment with different accessories and styles. Try wearing different kinds of earrings and find out how the wig looks with scarves, hats, and hair ornaments. On your own or with your wig stylist or a friend, try tying the wig back, or clip it to one side; add a couple of funky little braids, decorated with ribbons or beads. There are some excellent videotapes illustrating the different types of wigs that are available and showing how these wigs can be styled in different ways. These videos also demonstrate professional approaches to wearing and caring for wigs. Some companies that manufacture wigs make such videotapes available to their customers.

Most people who develop alopecia areata grab the first scarf or hat they can find that will cover their head while they try to cope with the situation. This is a natural response to losing your hair. Instead of sticking with that hat or scarf, though, you may want to buy a ready-made, inexpensive synthetic wig in a department store. For most women, we recommend this if the disease is affecting more than about 30 percent of the scalp hair. You can wear this wig while you continue to research the many other resources available to cover your head. Buying a wig at this point helps you realize that you *do* have choices in this area. That helps take some pressure off.

This particular wig and this time period can be considered a "trial run" during which you will begin to find out how wearing a wig fulfills your needs and fits your lifestyle. Wear this wig for two or three months, if possible, while you gather as much information as you can and prepare to buy the hairpiece that will really suit you. (You may decide that this wig does just fine, although that's un-likely.) A wig may be a major expense—the cost of a wig can range between $100 or less for a ready-made wig, all the way up to $3,000 or more for a state-of-the-art, top-quality hair replacement system—but it's going to have a great effect on your image and your self-esteem. Don't be in too much of a hurry. You wouldn't buy a new car on impulse without thinking through your needs, the price, the terms, the guarantees, and other factors involved in making a wise decision that you can live with.

To find out about wigs, ask your doctor or send away for information. You can visit wig salons, and you can talk to people who own wigs. It's also often very helpful to talk with hairstylists, who are very knowledgeable about wigs. Send away to as many different manufacturers as possible so you can see the full range of styles that are available, from casual and curly to sleek and sophisticated. Enlist the help of a good friend, partner, or parent in your search for information and in your decision making. You may also want to work with a wig consultant. If you want the truth, and the facts, rather than flattery, make this clear from the beginning to your advisor—whether kin, friend, or pro-fessional.

Wigs make us look different, the same as glasses or hats, so be prepared for a different look. A good approach is to tell yourself, "I'm going to look the best I can, and that's going to be a bit different from how I used to look and how I look now." People who forget this end up dis-appointed and sometimes feel robbed because they have spent so much time and money and don't look exactly like they used to. Wigs also make us *feel* different. They may cover up the "real you." The person who understands this and is open to the process of getting used to wearing a hairpiece and having a changed image, day after day, has the best chance of making the most of the situation and getting on with life.

No wig can bring back the past, but a wig can give you a chance to spruce up your appearance and look even more special. You might even look better than you ever did before your hair fell out. Not only do you have a choice of the most glamorous or dashing hairpieces, you can achieve a wonderful "do" in minutes rather than spending all that time washing it, drying it, moussing, gelling, and getting frustrated. Depending on how much money you spent on hair care in the past, you may also save a good bit of cash. (It's always useful to remember there *is* the odd advantage in losing hair.) Wigs give you a choice. They give you a certain freedom when your life seems limited by hair loss.

Wigs are a prosthesis, and they're also a sort of costume. They take some getting used to, and they take time and care and money—just like hair. Adjusting to your new hair, your new image, is a step-by-step process. Wearing your hairpiece will require both physical and psychological adjustment, and some serious thinking about your social life and how you deal with family and public situations as your new self with your new "hair." You may want to join an alopecia areata support group; the National Alopecia Areata Foundation can tell you about the one closest to you. Support groups provide a good forum for discussing the psychological aspects of wearing a wig.

They also often hold meetings where wigmakers demonstrate their wares, answer questions, and tell you everything you need to know about buying, fitting, styling, and maintenance.

Before continuing to describe the process of choosing and purchasing a wig, it's important to note that there are some methods of camouflaging hair loss that work fine for predictable, irreversible conditions such as androgenetic alopecia (pattern baldness, whether male or female) but that are definitely unsuitable for alopecia areata, where hair can regrow or fall out at any time. For people with alopecia areata, transplants are definitely not an option, since the expensive transplanted hair may fall out. Hair weaves or extensions are of value if the condition is stable. Since alopecia areata is usually not stable, these are not necessarily good options. And don't let anyone persuade you that surgically attached hairpieces will provide the perfect solution to your problem. They won't.

Wigs Work for Any Amount of Hair

If you have no hair, finding a wig that fits won't be a problem. Keeping it secure can be a problem, but one that is fading fast with improvements in technology. Years ago, as a teenager wearing a wig, I was walking home from school. A group of kids were throwing a hoola hoop around a fire hydrant. One of them threw it over my head, and it took my wig off. I picked the wig up, put it back on my head, and continued walking. (I wish I could have thought fast enough to say "good shot.") That won't happen to you if you do your homework and find the type of wig that will never fall off, no matter what. If you don't take the time to get a secure wig, you'd better make sure you cross the street when you see a hoola hoop.

If you have some hair, there are several options. You may decide to shave your remaining hair in order to achieve a close fit. You can do the same thing when your hair first begins to grow back, since shaving the hair that's there is less expensive than buying a new wig to fit your current amount of hair. If you have ever lost all your hair, you know how hard it would be to bring yourself to shave off the hair you have longed and prayed for. If you want to keep your hair, you can use it as a good base for fastening a wig to, but you'll probably need to buy a different wig.

As your hair grows longer and thicker and fuller, you might look for a full base supporting a partial hairpiece, blended and matched to complement your own hair. You can pull your own hair through the base to create a full head of hair. People with more hair than patches can select a smaller hairpiece or toupee and attach it with bobby pins, tape, clips, or decorative combs.

The simplest and cheapest cover-up for small bald patches is a soft lead eyebrow pencil. Find one that matches your hair color, and lightly "feather" the patch with small strokes to create the illusion of hair. A hairstylist can show you how to style your hair to soften the edge of the patch and partially cover it. Most people will never notice such a cunning disguise. Try out different types of eye pencils (waterproof, long-lasting, different brands and shades) until you find one that really fits the bill. A very effective cover-up for small or large patches is alopecia-masking lotion, usually found in a theatrical makeup store. It comes in a variety of colors and is easy to apply with a small sponge.

Wig Shopping

As noted above, you'll have to do some research before you begin to think about purchasing a wig that you'll want to wear for a long time. Ask the people in your support group or at the local chapter of the cancer society what salons and consultants they recommend. Some hospitals have on-site styling centers for people who have lost hair during treatment for cancer, and the staff in these centers may be particularly sensitive as well as knowledgeable.

Call around first, and have your friends and family make calls for you, before you begin visiting wig salons. You need to find out important information about the following:

- the wig company
- the facilities
- the wig
- wig maintenance

Once you've chosen the wig manufacturers or salons you wish to visit, it's a good idea to make an appointment with the consultant, so that he or she will clear some time in their schedule for showing you different wigs and talking with you about them.

If you are not naturally assertive—and who with alopecia has their assertiveness left intact?—it's useful to role-play with a friend or family member before you go to your appointment. You can practice asking the questions you want to ask and dealing with the consultant. Some consultants may try to evade your questions, and some may use hard-sell techniques; you'll want to be prepared for either of these possibilities—and be pleasantly surprised when neither occurs. Just knowing that you can handle yourself, no matter what happens, helps you to remain calm and composed in what can be an uncomfortable situation—being faced, once again, with your face in the mirror and the fact you have lost your hair.

It's also usually a good idea to take a friend or family member along—someone who is resourceful, assertive, supportive, and objective. Remember, however much your confidence has been affected by alopecia, that you are the customer, and you deserve good service. With hair loss, you may find it difficult to be assertive, which is why going with a friend can be helpful. There's safety in numbers. A friend can monitor whether you are trying to decide too quickly, or making what he or she thinks is a bad decision. Some merchants are hard sellers, so be prepared.

Now, here's what you should find out about *the company*. How long the company has been in business, and what qualifications and skills do the staff members have? Choose a wig consultant with whom you can talk easily on the phone, someone who appears to be understanding and who takes time to explain things to you. Ask for the names and telephone numbers of satisfied customers with whom you can talk about their experience with the company before you make an appointment. Find out how long the company takes to make a wig, or to receive shipment of a wig, what their wigs generally cost, and how long they are likely to last.

If you are ordering a custom-made wig, ask to see photographs of the same or a similar style on a client, or ask for the telephone number of a client with the same or similar style, so you can get in touch with the person and make arrangements to see for yourself. Most wig salons obtain permission from some of their clients to give out their phone number for this purpose. Ask to see a sample of the type of hairpiece you want to buy. Some wigmakers will try to get around this request with excuses, but don't be put off. Another thing you should ask is what makes this company's hairpieces better than their competitors'. Make sure that you describe your lifestyle and your personality to the consultant—a corporate executive has different needs from a teenager who wants to participate in sports. Also, someone who is shy may not want a hairpiece that is so glamorous that it draws comments from strangers, co-workers, or neighbors.

Be sure to find out whether the company can help you or advise you about filing a health insurance claim for a hairpiece (for this purpose, the better term to use is *cranial prosthesis;* see the appendix at the end of this book). Ask whether any of their customers have ever been successful in this. If so, this company may have some valuable tips to offer.

If you are buying an expensive, custom-made hairpiece, get the terms, the cost, and a warranty in writing. Find out whether the wig manufacturer has a money-back guarantee if the wig doesn't hold up under normal wear-and-care conditions; most reputable companies will provide some sort of guarantee, even if they prorate the refund, meaning that they will refund part of the cost but will deduct something for the time you've already had use of the wig.

When it comes to *the facilities,* what you're looking for is privacy, and mental as well as physical comfort. In private fitting rooms you can try on whatever you like without feeling uncomfortable, embarrassed, or panicked into buying the first wig you try on. If, when you telephone ahead for your appointment, you find out that no private room is available, ask the salesperson to arrange ahead of time for you to use a private washroom where you can try on several wigs without pressure.

If you prefer not to be seen buying a wig in your town, either visit a hair replacement specialist in another location or investigate the many companies that sell hairpieces by mail. They will send you catalogs to browse through, and if you are not satisfied with what you ordered, you can get a refund or try other styles. To be safe, it's a good idea to make certain the company has a return policy, and to have a copy of that policy in writing, either in the catalog or directly from the company. Mail-order wigs are often cheaper than wigs bought in stores.

The wig, of course, is what it's all about. You'll want to do everything you can to ensure your satisfaction with your purchase. For starters, make certain that you can try on a variety of styles and colors. Ask whether the wigs are made from synthetic or real hair, and whether they are mass-produced or custom-made and custom-fitted. Find out what type of base the wig has.

Wig maintenance can be either a pain or relatively painless. As part of your telephone research, ask the consultant to describe the details of guarantees or warranties provided for the company's hairpieces, and to tell you what you can expect to invest in both time and money for maintenance, cleaning, restyling, and repairing. Whatever kind of wig you wear, treat your wig as carefully as you would treat expensive contact lenses. Follow the manufacturer's instructions for care precisely, and don't use anything on your wig other than what's recommended. The manufacturer or the salon consultant will tell you what type of brush or comb, cleaning solution, and styling procedures are recommended for the type of wig you purchase. These wig issues will be discussed more below.

Different Types of Hairpieces

You'll be able to make a good decision in buying a wig once you can answer the following questions. Keep doing your wig research until you're satisfied with your answers.

1. Do you want a ready-made, mass-produced wig (priced beginning at $50) or a custom-made one (which will be more expensive)?
2. Would you prefer synthetic hair or real (human) hair?
3. What type of attachment is right for you: stretch base with hook, tape or clips, or suction base?

READY-MADE OR CUSTOM-MADE?

Ready-made wigs are usually composed of synthetic materials, whereas custom-made wigs can be either synthetic or human hair or a combination; custom-made wigs also provide the widest range of attachment methods. Ready-made wigs are available from department stores, hair salons, and special wig stores as well as by mail order. Custom-made wigs are available from specialist wigmakers or hair replacement establishments, and by mail order.

Buy a ready-made wig at the first sign of significant hair loss. These wigs adjust to most head sizes, and they are so reasonably priced that you can afford to make mistakes, upgrade, or buy a few to play with, especially if you like being outrageous from time to time. A good hairstylist can also make a ready-made piece look more natural by thinning and styling it.

Once they get used to wearing a wig, many people with alopecia areata order a custom-made hairpiece. Whether purchased through a mail-order company or at a salon, custom-made wigs can be dyed to match exactly any remaining hair. They can also be designed to fit your age and your lifestyle. It often looks more natural for someone who is over age forty, say, to have a little gray in their hair or a slightly receding hairline than to have the thickness and brilliance of a teenage head of hair. Custom-made wigs are usually hand-knotted onto the base (again, this can create a more natural hairline than ready-made wigs usually have). Because of the labor involved, hand-knotted hairpieces are more expensive.

Custom-made wigs must be personally fitted. The normal procedure is for a mold to be made of your head, either by you or the consultant, with kitchen plastic wrap and tape. This mold is marked with the hairline that will suit your face, then usually sent away to the factory where the wig is made. Expect to wait a few weeks for the finished product, which will then be fitted to your head and styled by a professional. If you are ordering by mail, you will have to take your head measurements yourself, but the company will provide clear instructions how to do this. They may also recommend a local hair salon where you can have your new "hair" styled to suit.

SYNTHETIC OR HUMAN HAIR?

Acrylic and other synthetic fibers are the most practical. They can provide a lightweight, stylish, natural look compared with the stiff shiny wigs of a few years ago, and they last for years. Normally these wigs can be cared for at home: wash them, place them on a wig stand to keep the shape, and let them dry. If they get wet, take them off carefully at home and dry them. They dry more quickly and with less tangling than human hair. Synthetic wigs are the best bet when it comes to children (for more information about buying a wig for a child, see chapter 5).

Synthetic wigs do have certain drawbacks, though. The fibers used in some of the wigs look unnaturally shiny, so be sure to shop around. Another disadvantage of synthetic wigs is that if you style them, the style will not last as long as on human hair. Sleeping in them can spoil their appearance. Acrylic wigs can be ruined by heat, which melts the fibers. Never wear an acrylic wig into a sauna or when looking into the oven to check on your cooking.

Unlike synthetics, wigs made from human hair look and feel completely natural. They can also be styled like real hair, so you aren't stuck with the same old style month after month. Like real hair, with a human hair wig, you can use mousse, gel, and lotions to style it, and you can perm or color it. You can have as much variety in your hairstyle as you have ever had before. Unfortunately, these wigs do not last as long as synthetics—about a year or two, depending on how conscientiously they are cared for. That's because once the hair is cut from its donor, it gradually loses its beauty as it oxidizes (changes shade to redder or yellower) with exposure to air and sun. After all, it's real hair and it behaves like real hair.

People who are active in sports are harder on human hair wigs, because of all that fresh air and sun and water. European hair is the finest, but Oriental hair is tougher and can be treated in more ways. Real hair is more expensive than synthetic, but the difference may be worth it. It's your choice. A few companies offer wigs that are a blend of human and synthetic fibers. Be sure to check carefully about maintenance and potential problems, because the two fibers are so different that you could end up with an unmanageable mess.

SECURING THE WIG

The base to which the hair is attached is a very important part of any wig. Although you will read that the manufacturer has an exclusive, even patented, base or attachment, all attachments are variations on three main types: stretch base with hook, tape or clips, and suction base. The simplest is a structured, often stretchy net (or other open-weave) base that fastens together with a small hook to make the wig fit your head—much like an elasticized waistband.

Wigs can also be attached by means of double-sided surgical adhesive tape, Velcro or small clips attached to a cap worn fitting very close to the head. The tape or Velcro is sewn inside the hairpiece at several strategic points and then attached to an oiled silk patch worn close to the head. Wigs can be both clipped and taped for ultimate security, which avoids any problems with the tape losing its stick in extreme cold or when perspiring heavily.

For greatest security, the more expensive option is a base that holds to the head by suction or vacuum. With this kind of wig, the suction cup is molded to fit your head by a special process. When the wig is completed, it attaches to your head with a vacuum seal—similar to what happens when you put a lid on a piece of Tupperware. And even though it will stay on when you go swimming or engage in active sports, it can be removed easily, too—again, much like a Tupperware lid. The hairpiece is very light-weight and comfortable, and it doesn't overheat. Not every salon carries these systems, however. If you have trouble finding a salon that does, you can call the National Alopecia Areata Foundation (see Resources), which will provide a list of suppliers as well as information about support groups in your area, whose members may know where you can find a vendor nearby.

Whatever the method of fastening, a separate patch

or cap worn beneath the wig—sometimes called a liner—provides extra security and comfort. These caps are made of breathable material, such as PVC or fiberglass, to prevent the scalp from overheating. Other light, cool bases are made of thin silk, nylon, or lace.

If you have only small patches to cover, you may want to use a hair "add-on." Add-ons are lengths of hair that attach to your own hair; you can buy add-ons in a color close to your own, or you can dye them to match your own hair. For a perfect match, dye both the add-on and your own hair. Some add-ons are simply clipped to your own hair; others come glued to decorative combs that you just place in your hair wherever they're needed. Some wig manufacturers offer hairpieces that can be attached to wide headbands in a range of colors to wear with different outfits.

Some salons offer hairpieces that can be glued to the head with solutions that dissolve into the scalp but retain the bond. They stick, but you're stuck with them, literally, for weeks until you return to the salon to have the bond professionally dissolved. Cleaning and hygiene are tricky, and if the wig gets caught, your scalp gets pulled, and it hurts. Rarely, the glue can irritate your skin and can cause an allergic reaction.

Choosing a Style

Your first, inexpensive, wig should help you decide what you really want when you upgrade, in terms of weight, comfort, and realism (including color). Just as you do when you try on clothes, check out how the wig looks in natural light by looking in a mirror while you stand at a window in the salon. Colors look different in fluorescent light. Consider your facial shape and skin coloring, rather than trying to match your own hair or falling for the color and style of your wildest dreams. It may look good, but does it look good on *you?*

Something in the way of bangs or wavy style softens the hairline and helps disguise that you are wearing a hairpiece. A common mistake at the selection stage is opting for a hairline that is too low. Some people want to hide behind a hairline that starts too low on the forehead, perhaps trying to conceal missing eyebrows or lashes. Instead, you want to make a decision based on the quality and naturalness of the style, not the quantity of hair in the piece.

If you're in doubt about where your hairline should be, pay attention for a while to where other people's hairlines fall, before you order your wig. Notice other people's hair as you walk down the street or around the mall, and how the hair looks around the ears and back of head, too. Ask your friend to check the side and back of the neck when you are trying on wigs. Does it look natural, or does it appear to be stuck on over the skin? Does the hairline go straight across, like a bowl cut? Ask your friends how your wig looks. Good friends tell you if you have raspberry seeds stuck in your teeth. You can count on them to tell you in a caring way how your wig looks.

Another point to check is whether the wig has too much hair—difficult to resist when you have too little. If you've lost your hair, your instinct may be to cover your scalp with as much hair as possible. Wigs are generally thicker than your own hair, but *too much hair* often looks unnatural and may not suit your face. A stylist can thin the wig so that it looks more natural. Although you may feel as if, once again, you are being deprived of hair, your aim is to look natural and unobtrusive, not like you've won the big hair stakes. Men have to pay particular attention to the volume of the hairpiece; to obtain a natural appearance you may have to opt for slightly thinner hair than you'd like, rather than going for the werewolf "rug."

Another thing to consider when you're tempted to go for a huge volume of hair is the comfort factor. Weight has to be a consideration in making your purchase. Walk around with the wig on, and move about and see how it feels after several minutes. That glamorous Cher-style fall of curls may give you a pain in the neck after an hour or two.

Some hair salons provide computer technology as a service to their customers (at a cost), so they can see how various cuts and colors will look on their actual faces. If your hair replacement salon offers this service, take the time and spend the money to use it, because it will allow you to consider carefully what you are prepared to live with. Computer technology can generate pictures of you in different hairstyles, so you can avoid the hair disaster of going for a style that looks great on an elfin-faced model but very odd indeed with your own classical features, or a color that's too vibrant or that doesn't complement your skin tone in some other way.

Computer imaging is invaluable for seeing the kind of

look you may want before deciding what kind of wig to buy. To use this service, you won't have to remove any hairpiece that you're currently wearing. What happens is that the stylist takes a picture of you, then alters it on the computer to remove all hair from the image; they do the same thing with pictures of people who have their own hair. You then go through a book with a stylist and select from a huge variety of colors—about seventy-two thousand—and from up to two hundred hairstyles. The computer produces an image of your face wearing hair in the color and style of your choice. At a typical salon, less than fifty dollars will buy you an hour of computer imaging. You make twelve selections (style and color) and view them; decide which four you like best, and go home with a color print of your four favorites to muse upon and gather responses from friends and family. Then, when you go to buy your hairpiece, you *know* that what you envision and what your dealer and stylist thinks you see are the same—she or he has the picture.

A perfect-looking head of hair may look perfect, or it may look a little artificial, like wearing obviously perfect makeup. Do you want to go for the look of perfection? Or will you mistreat your wig a little, ruffle it, and let it get slightly messy and dull, so that it looks like a real head of hair on a "bad hair" day? The choice is yours, and it really depends on your wardrobe, your image, your lifestyle—and *you.* Whatever type of wig and fastening you choose, take the time to make sure that you've put it on the right way before dashing out the door!

Wig Care

Wigs are easier to maintain than real hair. You don't have to cut them regularly, or be an expert stylist to look good. You just take them off, shake them out, and voilà! they look exactly the same day after day. More expensive wigs, particularly the human hair type, require more care. If you've spent that much money to look good, don't mess up the effect by skimping on maintenance. When the wig begins to look matted or straggly, or if the color has strayed too far from the original, take the wig back to the salon (or send it to the manufacturer) for cleaning. The wig can be redyed if the hair has oxidized, and individual hairs that have come loose can be retied.

Wigs don't last forever: like items of clothing or shoes, they go through various stages and eventually wear out. In other words, you can't buy a lifetime guarantee for your wig. On the other end of the process, it's important to note that you're not likely to find that your wig "fits" exactly right in the very beginning. Also like shoes, wigs take some "breaking in." This process may take two or three months. You will need time to get used to it, and your wig will need time to "weather" a little and look more natural.

After about six months of constant wear, a wig begins to lose its shape, especially if it's the kind that has a stretchy base. It's important to purchase a new wig before the old one needs replacing, so you can generally count on purchasing a new wig annually. Most people have a "spare" wig that they wear either for special occasions or for grocery shopping and yard work; switching off like this will extend, maybe even double, the life of both wigs, because they can "rest" in between wearings. If you have a spare wig, too, you'll never be stuck if one of your wigs needs to be sent for repair, cleaning, or restyling—or if it has an accident of any kind.

Health Insurance Reimbursement for Wigs

In addition to coping with psychological and social adjustments, people with alopecia areata often experience financial difficulties because of the cost of medical treatment and hairpieces or other cover-ups. Thanks to the determination of patients, doctors, and the National Alopecia Areata Foundation—and encouragement from hair replacement professionals—in pursuing reimbursement, health insurance companies and health care administrators and legislators are becoming more familiar with alopecia areata.

Hairpieces are essential for most people, and they can be expensive. Nevertheless, it often takes great persistence to recover the cost of a hairpiece from your medical insurance. While pursuing expense claims can be frustrating, many people report that doing so gives them a great sense of achievement. The important reasons to keep on trying are for your own mental and financial betterment and also because many small victories improve the situation for everyone who has alopecia areata.

What seems most unfair is that people with temporary alopecia due to cancer treatments have their hairpiece costs reimbursed, while those of us who have to live for months or years with hair loss usually have to pay for our wigs

ourselves. Why the disparity? Until recently there was little awareness of alopecia areata even in many medical cir-
cles, even less among health care administrators and insurance companies. Part of the problem lies in terminology.

When a part of the body is lost through surgery or disease, it can sometimes be replaced with an artificial part
known as a *prosthesis* (plural *prostheses*), which maintains
the function of the missing part. Thus what used to be known
as a false leg is now called a prosthesis: the prosthesis
allows the person to walk and to look fairly normal. A
woman whose breast is removed as part of her treatment
for cancer usually wears a breast prosthesis to maintain
the appearance of normality—the prosthesis allows her to
function as a social being without comments or stares.

A wig, on the other hand, has always been regarded as
a cosmetic device—something worn purely for appearance's sake. However, it is now becoming clear that alopecia areata may severely limit not just social and psychological functioning, but also the person's ability to
function in society, at school or at work. Indeed, it may be
expected in some jobs that a wig must be worn. In such
cases, a hairpiece is not just a cosmetic, it is clearly an essential, as the American Academy of Dermatology White
Paper on alopecia areata states: "The disease . . . represents
a grave challenge to the functional status of the patient
and it is not possible to lead a productive, normal life without a suitable full cranial prosthesis. The need for a full
cranial prosthesis is much the same as the need for a leg
prosthesis by someone with an amputated leg."

Filing a Claim with Your Insurer

Different states in the United States and different provinces in Canada have enacted different legislation about hairpieces. At present, some insurance carriers and health maintenance organizations (HMOs) in the United States cover treatment and hairpiece costs for patients with alopecia areata, and some do not. In Canada, visits to doctors and dermatologists are covered under the provincial medical plans, but patients have to pay the cost of drugs or chemicals used in treatment, unless the treatment is part of a clinical study. This disparate situation is made more confusing by the proliferation of insurance carriers and health plan providers. It is not helped by the fact that in some states, legislation has been passed to award reimbursement to patients with alopecia areata, while in other states and at the federal level the issue has not been clarified. Some insurance companies provide full reimbursement, some partial, others none at all.

Minnesota, for example, passed legislation in August 1987 requiring all insurance carriers, including HMOs to pay up to $350 per annum toward the cost of hairpieces. New Hampshire passed similar legislation in January 1993. At the federal level, House Bill 4872—an act providing health insurance coverage for scalp hair prostheses—is currently stalled.

People with alopecia areata who have extended medical insurance are in the best position. Treatment for the condition is usually covered, and all or part of the cost of a hairpiece is generally reimbursed, especially when the claim is accompanied by supporting documents such as letters from a dermatologist, a psychiatrist or psychologist, or a social worker, as well as a copy of the AAD White Paper and any magazine or newspaper articles that document the trauma caused by alopecia areata. In Canada, up to $1,400 may be claimed during a two-year period through extended medical coverage—but patients may have to fight for the coverage. Some patients in Canada claim the cost of their cranial prosthesis as a tax deduction: if an individual's medical costs are greater than 3 percent of their income, they may do so. Health care services and health care funding are currently under review both in the United States and in many Canadian provinces. Therefore, we suggest that you check with NAAF, wig suppliers, or insurance companies for updated information on legislation and insurance practices.

People who have no health insurance or who are not able to obtain reimbursement under their present policy may need to think creatively about other sources of funding. You may want to contact cancer clinics for information about resources for funding such as foundations or community groups.

The National Alopecia Areata Foundation recommends that patients with health insurance who live in the United States follow these procedures to obtain reimbursement:

- File a claim
- Prepare for the claim to be denied
- Consider taking the case to a small claims court

To make your claim for reimbursement as strong as possible, take the following steps:

- Find out what your medical plan covers by reading your policy carefully, particularly any sections that mention "prosthesis" or "prosthetic device." Be prepared to cite the provisions of your plan to a representative from the insurance company.
- Include a cover letter from your dermatologist or family doctor that mentions "scalp or cranial prosthesis" (see sample letters in the appendix). Include a copy of the American Academy of Dermatology White Paper on Alopecia Areata. You can obtain a copy from the Department of Socioeconomic and Practice Issues, AAD, 930 N. Meacham Road, P.O. Box 4014, Schaumburg, IL 60164–4014.
- Include a receipt from the person who manufactured or sold you your hairpiece. The receipt must include the magic phrase "scalp or cranial prosthesis." Make sure that it is signed and dated by the wig manufacturer or merchant.

Additional convincing evidence for the decision-making bodies may include:

- A photograph of yourself without any hairpiece, false eyelashes, or makeup. You may not like the look of it, but it will convey to them the reality of how you look without this "prosthesis."
- A photograph of yourself before you lost hair. This will illustrate the change you have to cope with.

- A letter from an employer or mental health professional detailing the importance of "hair" for your job
and your mental health and social functioning. Such a
letter can be very persuasive.

To get you started, sample letters to insurance companies seeking benefits for "cranial prostheses" are provided
in the appendix. You will be in the best position if your
policy states that you have coverage and if you clearly document the need for the wig, as described above. If your
coverage is not clear in this area and if your claim is refused, it doesn't hurt to file again. And again. It's possible
that the insurance company will tire of the claim and simply put it through.

To help change the situation for all of us, you may
want to contact your state or provincial insurance com-
missioner and try to get legislation changed in your state
or province, using the resources of your support group.
By working together to establish precedents and change
legislation, we can all benefit and make the financial side
of alopecia areata easier for ourselves and future generations.

Getting Used to Wearing a Wig

ADJUSTING PHYSICALLY

When you wear a wig, you need to remain alert to situations that can cause problems: clothing snagging your
hair, people brushing past you, windy days, people hugging you. You can usually see a hug coming and take eva-
sive action of some sort. In a theater or on public trans-

portation, you'll need to be aware of people's movements and incline your head out of the way if it looks like they're going to come into physical contact with you. You also must be careful getting out of a car so that your wig doesn't get caught on the roof. You need to be alert to the possibility of people touching your hair, whether it's a date wanting to run his or her fingers through your lovely tresses, a jovial fellow worker, or a playful child or baby. You may have to ask them not to touch your hair; if you don't want to say that you wear a wig, you can just say that it makes you uncomfortable to have your hair touched.

When you wear a wig, you also have to think more about the kind of clothing you wear. Cardigan sweaters and shirts or blouses that zip or button up will not dislodge your wig, while those that have to be pulled on or off over the head may. Also, wearing a hairpiece usually makes people hotter than they would be with their own hair, so you may perspire more. Consider this in selecting your outfit.

Wearing a wig in bed may be essential for both adults and children, depending on who else is sleeping in the same bedroom. Wigs require a greater awareness of how you move about while sleeping, and possibly an early morning check in the bathroom for grooming. Wigs can also be comfortable at night, if your head gets cold. Or you may want to choose a soft cotton jersey headcover for comfort or a woolly cap in winter to keep your head warm.

In time you'll become more relaxed about wearing a wig. Whether you resent having to wear a hairpiece or not, treat your hairpiece with respect. It's part of your image. You are caring for yourself and your extended self.

ADJUSTING PSYCHOLOGICALLY

The best way to get used to this new part of you is to practice wearing your wig. Wear it at home before you ever wear it out, so you get used to how you look, with the feel of it, and with any mannerisms or situations that may interfere with it. Just as with contact lenses, glasses, or dentures, it will take some time for you to adjust to wearing a hairpiece, time for it to feel like part of you and not like an attachment. Then wearing it in public will be much easier, and you can take it in your stride. Just like with contacts, you will forget it's there.

INTIMATE RELATIONSHIPS

There are no rules for coping with a wig during intimate moments. You will have to work out what's best for you and for those closest to you, depending on your attitudes and sensitivities—and theirs. Having sex while wearing a wig is a challenge, there's no question about it. Many people with alopecia areata go through a period of avoiding physical contact because their date doesn't know about their wig. After all, if your wig slips during a passionate moment, it can destroy the atmosphere and cause great embarrassment.

When you're going to become intimate with someone, it's usually best to tell that person that you wear a wig. Of course, if you already have a partner when you lose your hair, both of you will need to get used to your wearing a wig. Many people become comfortable without a wig. If you meet someone after your hair has fallen out, and if you want to be close to your new partner, you need to let him or her know that you wear a hairpiece, however difficult that may be. This does *not* mean you have to let the other person see you without your wig, if that makes you (or him or her) anxious or uncomfortable. Simply let the person know that you wear a prosthesis. Say, "I wear a wig." Don't keep it secret and pretend that you have a full head of hair, because sooner or later the other person will either suspect or find out, and that is harder to cope with than having the person know what is going on in the first place. Whenever intimacy between two people is involved, the more honest you are, the easier it will be in the long run.

Most people respond very supportively when they are told that their partner wears a wig, although some people are insensitive or embarrassed, and they may act or speak inappropriately. If your date accepts your hair loss, hold onto him or her. If he or she doesn't—if he comments on it frequently or she jokes insensitively or if they believe you aren't a "real" man or woman without hair—you will need to ask yourself whether you really want to develop a deep relationship with such a person.

Even supportive partners may find it difficult to accept that you need to wear a wig, so you may not want to leave your wig lying around. It may make life much easier if you simply treat your wig like a set of dentures. You wouldn't leave dentures lying around to remind your nearest and dearest of your lack of teeth. Most women don't leave their bras or nylons hanging around for others to see, either. Unless you're certain that having your wigs on display is not a problem, you may want to keep them in a cabinet. This will also keep them safe from toddlers and pets.

SPORTS

It used to be that people with wigs avoided certain sports because their hairpieces were unreliable and they didn't want to risk the embarrassment of having them fall off. Today, there are hairpieces that hold so firmly, and work so well in water and sun and rain, that people with alopecia areata can participate in aerobics, swim, snow ski, and water ski with confidence and enjoyment. You do not have to limit yourself. Given the health and psychological benefits of physical fitness and sports, don't give in to the feeling that all that's left for you is staying at home and doing exercise videos on your own.

THE GREAT DEBATE: WHO NEEDS TO KNOW?

To tell or not to tell: That's the "big" question. Now, most people wouldn't march around the office or shop telling people that they wear dentures or have had cosmetic surgery. And who goes around showing off their hearing aids? Likewise, if you don't want to, you don't have to tell anyone that you wear a wig. It's nobody's business but your own.

On the other hand, once you have become used to wearing your "hair," you may find you would rather not keep your secret from absolutely everybody. Disclosing your secret will allow you to experience acceptance from other people, which in turn increases your self-esteem. There are many layers of people in your life, and it is your decision whom to tell—and when and how to tell them.

Sheila Jacobs, author of *The Big Fall: Living with Hair Loss,* seldom wears wigs or hats. She once encountered a wig problem in reverse, though, while applying for a place in an educational program. That day Sheila wore her wig in order to make a good impression and keep the interview focused on her application rather than her head. But when she arrived, she found that her interviewer was someone she knew as the president of her local residents' association.

"Don't I know you?" he asked, puzzled.
"Yes, it's Sheila, but I'm wearing my wig today because of coming to this interview."

Sheila says that the lecturer seemed quite embarrassed, and she herself didn't know whether to whip off the wig and reveal the head he knew, or keep it on and pretend this was just a normal, everyday exchange. She kept the wig on—and was accepted into the program.

Eyelashes and Eyebrows

Eyelashes protect our eyes, and eyebrows do that as well as help to shape our facial expressions. Eyelashes and eyebrows are small but important parts of the human face, and for people who lose them, there's a need to compensate for their loss in some way. For women this is easier than for men, since women can use makeup and wear false eyelashes, if they want.

It's not generally acceptable for men to wear facial makeup, so they have a more difficult time trying to disguise a lack of eyebrows and lashes. As noted above, wearing a hairpiece low on the forehead with thick bangs in an attempt to cover the eyebrow area might only draw more attention to your "hair." A better option for men might be wearing glasses, with plain glass if you have no ophthalmologic need for them; eyeglass frames can partially camouflage the lack of eyebrows and distract attention away from a lack of eyelashes. Tinted glasses provide a light disguise that still allows eye-to-eye contact. If patches appear in a man's beard they can be shaded with pencils or camouflage cream, but the easiest solution is to shave the beard off altogether.

For women, a feathering technique of applying make-up in the eyebrow area works well for missing or partially missing eyebrows, and looks more natural than crayoning on an eyebrow-shaped outline and coloring it in. A light touch with an eyebrow pencil or a cake eyeliner with a fine brush is best. Try a shade *lighter* than your original brow color; a common mistake is to choose a color that is too dark and looks artificial. Better still, use two or more shades, since real hair is never just one shade, even on your brows. Try dabbing hairspray on eyebrows to set them in place so they don't smudge.

False eyelashes can overwhelm a face, so try the smallest, most insignificant ones you can find. Save the big, bold ones for a fancy evening out when you really want to look dramatic. Many women with alopecia areata find that a soft kohl pencil around the eye, smudged at the outer edges, provides the illusion of lashes, and it's quick and easy to apply.

Ask a good friend to help you achieve the most realistic look, or watch a videotape on the subject. If you belong to a support group, suggest that the group hold a makeup evening and invite a professional makeup artist to demonstrate. Cancer clinics can put you in touch with cosmetics professionals, such as the Look Good Feel Good organization, who are skilled at disguising lack of eyebrows and eyelashes.

Some companies offer to apply permanent eyebrows or "eyeliner" around the eyes, using a sophisticated method that results in a tattoo. This method provides permanent, smudge-proof, and waterproof color, though not the texture of hair. The technique has not been around long enough to know what the effects will be after years of having the color in place, as the skin naturally loses its elasticity and changes in other ways. Also, as we age our facial hair naturally begins to contain gray or white hairs; how will that dark color look when we should be showing our age in our facial hair? It is also unclear whether the person's appearance will be acceptable if, as happens to many people with alopecia areata, the eyebrows and lashes regrow, fully or partially.

If you choose this option, make sure that you find a reputable company. Again, like with buying a wig, ask for the names and telephone numbers of satisfied customers and go and see the results for yourself. There is no way of guaranteeing that there won't be any problems. The only way to remove a tattoo is with laser surgery. This procedure is very expensive and has a very low chance of resulting in scarring.

Scarves and Hats

The first cover-up for many people with alopecia areata is a scarf—any old scarf. Or some old baseball cap.

You're panicking, you fling it on, and no one can see you're patchy or thinning. After that initial response, however, you may never want to wear a scarf or cap again, once you find a wig that looks more "normal." But scarves come in so many beautiful fabrics and patterns, and they can be tied, wrapped, braided, and woven (alone or in pairs) in so many ways, that they can be a wonderful part of any wardrobe. And of course both scarves and hats are much cheaper than wigs, and they require less care. Bandannas are currently popular among teens and young adults, with or without hair.

Some companies that manufacture scarves and hats for people with less hair also sell little quilted jersey pads that add bulk, thereby providing the suggestion that hair lies beneath the scarf. Practice in front of the mirror, and consult with a friend. Your local cancer agency may have videotapes demonstrating the use of scarves.

Hats are hot fashion items these days. You can find a huge variety of hats in department stores and specialist hat shops, and you can get hats through the mail, as well, from companies that specialize in cover-ups for people losing hair. Some creations are of structured cotton-mix jersey that combine the comfort of scarves with the ease and style of hats. Many can be dressed up or down, and some are available with contrast scarves or headbands. They are the most comfortable option for sleeping in, and they keep the head warm on cold nights.

Stores that sell wigs often have a selection of scarves, soft hats, and accessories that the storekeepers can arrange or combine in stylish and creative ways for you. Turbans are always popular for beach or leisure wear, or for swimming, especially in cool and easy-care terry cloth or glamorous velour. A favorite for people with alopecia areata, especially men, kids, and outdoor types, is the baseball cap. Anyone can make a fashion statement in the kind of velvet, sequined caps available now.

One particularly versatile creation is the hat or scarf that has a section of "hair" sewn to it. Sometimes the pieces are interchangeable: you can buy three different styles or colors of caps and simply fit the hair into whichever one you are wearing. To avoid that hairless hat look, you can have a softly gathered cap with bangs, or a straw hat with a couple of inches of "hair" sewn around the sides and back. Alternatively, buy your own hairpieces and attach them yourself to your favorite headcoverings. It's time to get creative! Wearing a scarf or turban under a hat can look so dramatic and attractive that no one will even notice that no hair is visible. And clips, jeweled pins, and other accessories can dress a hat or scarf up or down according to your mood.

Questions to Ask Yourself

Finally, here are some questions to ask yourself when you're deciding what you want to do when it comes to hairpieces and headcoverings. In making this decision, you need to consider your appearance, your personality, and your lifestyle:

- What are your needs and wishes?
- What activities do you want to continue?
- Do you want a complete change of image, or something that looks similar to your own hair?

- How much time, effort, and money, do you want to spend on this part of your life?

When you've answered these questions, you'll have a very good idea about what kinds of cover-ups are going to work for you.

FIVE

Special Considerations for Children

The parents of a little girl with alopecia areata
bought her a wig when she said that she wanted to
have her "own" hair. But the little girl didn't want
to wear the wig, she just wanted to keep it at home
in her room. When a stranger asked her one day
what had happened to her hair, she smiled and said,
"Oh, I left it at home."

The lifetime risk of developing alopecia areata for any
healthy child is extremely low. Seventeen people in a thousand, or 1.7 percent of all people, will develop alopecia
areata. Even for children with a parent who has the disease, only 6 percent will get the disease. And only 2 percent of all children born to a parent with alopecia areata
will have severe disease. But for any child with a disease,
especially one like alopecia areata which is so visible, the
already bumpy road of childhood can be even more difficult to travel.

Children have something going for them when it comes
to dealing with the bumps in the road of life, though, and
that is that they are amazingly resilient. Most children,
like the little girl described above, are creative problem-
solvers. Nevertheless, a child who begins losing hair and
then is diagnosed with alopecia areata needs special help
in dealing with this condition and the changes that it
brings. Parents and siblings as well as doctors and teach-

ers can help make the child's life less stressful by being honest about the condition and by following the child's or adolescent's lead in deciding how, and how aggressively, to deal with it.

There are, of course, vast differences between toddlers and teenagers, and decisions about how to handle alopecia areata have to take into account these life-stage differences as well as the more personal differences between individual children. A child's age and life-stage have a huge effect on how he or she deals with alopecia. Preschoolers are usually more interested in making sense of and experimenting with the physical world than in paying attention to the details of people's appearances, including their own. When they do notice that someone looks different they're usually fascinated, but they seldom label such differences as being wrong, bad, or "abnormal."

In elementary school, children begin learning about social expectations. They may focus on similarities and differences and begin to make scapegoats of those who look or speak differently. By the age of thirteen or fourteen, children begin to realize they can affect how their friends feel, for better or worse, and in the years that follow they tend to start being more careful of each others' feelings. But the teenage years are also a time of tremendous physical and emotional change, and they may be especially difficult years for the child with alopecia areata.

Feelings

Children with alopecia areata face big challenges. They have to incorporate their hair loss into a self-identity that's still in the formative stage. They have to deal with interruptions for frequent doctor visits and the nuisance of medications and discomfort of other treatments. They have to agonize over whether they can take part in activities like tumbling, gymnastics, and swimming, weighing their desire to do so against their fear of losing their head covering. They have to balance the hope that their hair will grow back with the reality of the situation as it exists now. But without doubt, the most difficult challenge for children with alopecia areata is how other children react to them.

At a certain age, many children can't seem to pass up the opportunity to make a big deal out of anyone who looks different. They might call a little girl who has no hair a "boy" because she wears a baseball cap all the time. Depending upon how the child reacts as well as the nature and socialization of the children doing the teasing, they may let it go at that, or they may escalate the teasing. It may become really vicious, and the child being teased may be not just hurt, but traumatized. One eight-year-old boy was picked on and teased so much that he became withdrawn; because of this, his teachers decided that he wasn't ready to move on to the next grade in school, and they held him back—which meant that he had to face another classroom full of strangers the next year.

Being teased and called names like "baldy," having your hat or wig ripped off—or being chased by someone who is threatening to do so—can be traumatic. There's no question that children hurt when they're teased, and so do their parents. The solution to this problem involves a three-pronged approach. The first is to equip children with an effective defense: information, words, and attitudes that

they can use to feel good about themselves and to decrease
the teasing or stop it altogether. The second is to educate
the children who are doing the teasing; their entire attitude may change if they understand *why* the other child
has no hair or has to wear a hat or a wig. Finally, it's often
necessary to teach the adults who interact with the child
who has alopecia areata *about* alopecia areata; this includes
teachers, principals, school nurses, and lunchroom workers as well as family members, friends, and neighbors outside of the school setting.

If your child has alopecia areata, you need to explain
to the child why his or her hair is falling out and what the
prognosis is. Children have their own view of the world
and active imaginations, and they'll come up with all sorts
of things on their own if they're not kept well informed.
As we mentioned in chapter 2, a big part of coping is understanding, so you will want to make sure that your child
understands. Depending on your child's age, you can say
something like this:

> Alopecia areata is like an allergy to your hair. It won't
> hurt. It is not contagious, or "catching," and otherwise
> you are perfectly healthy. You don't have cancer, and
> doctors aren't sure yet what causes your hair to fall out.
> It is not your fault, and you haven't done anything
> wrong. There is nothing wrong with you, you just look
> different. The doctor is going to work with us to try to
> find a treatment that will make your hair grow back.

Once your child understands these things about the condition, he or she will probably be better able to put up a
good defense against bullies. Children who learn to stand

their ground and verbally confront a bully may accomplish two things: they may stop the teasing and simultaneously strengthen their own self-respect.

Sometimes the best defense for children who are being teased is the timely and proper delivery of a few well-practiced "wisecracks." Parents and other adults can help the child practice these responses to teasing, and to stand up for themselves and—if necessary—to fight back with words, instead of swallowing what bullies say to them. It's not a nice game to have to play, but the child's emotional score will be higher if clever retorts are used instead of responses that reveal anger or hurt. Mean words are hard to digest, and it's not a good idea to eat them.

For the second prong in dealing with the problem of teasing, it's necessary to educate the other children about alopecia areata. One important caveat is that this approach should not be used without the knowledge and, in most cases, the consent of the child with the condition. For children who cope with alopecia areata by denying that there is a problem, and children who just don't want anyone to talk about it, this approach may not be appropriate. Parents can point out the advantages of talking with the other children, but it is never appropriate to force the child to agree to this approach—or to talk with the other children "behind the child's back." On the other hand, many children find it easier to be open about their hair loss than to keep it a secret, and they will usually be glad to have their classmates understand better what's going on with them. That way they have nothing to hide and can go about their business, letting go of their anxiety about being "discovered."

To teach the other children about alopecia areata, parents may want to arrange to talk to the children in the classroom, or to work through the teacher, who can integrate a presentation on alopecia areata into the rest of the classwork (the teacher may have to learn about the condition, too). The parent or the teacher who is teaching the children about alopecia can say something similar to what was suggested above. Another option is to ask the doctor, nurse, or social worker to make a presentation to the class, to demystify the condition. The child with alopecia areata should be the one who decides whether he or she will be there when the presentation takes place.

How do we know that it helps to educate the child's classmates and other peers about alopecia areata? This approach has proven useful time and again for children who are returning to school after a disfiguring injury such as a burn or an amputation. In fact, many hospitals and burn centers have developed school reentry programs where the health care team go into the classroom and prepare classmates for what's different about the child who is coming back to school. When it's appropriate, they use special puppets to show children what they can expect when they see their classmate again. Taking the mystery and fear out of the physical difference, and approaching it in a matter-of-fact way, often means that kids are prepared and willing, even glad, to welcome their pal comfortably back into the group.

While parents should avoid being overprotective, it's natural for them to want to protect their child from harm, including emotional hurt. In a teasing situation, parents sometimes become so upset at their child's tormenters that they rush in and scold the other children, to punish them and try to get them to stop. Unfortunately, this is seldom a successful way to solve the problem. On the other hand, if your child gives the okay, you can calmly remind other children that teasing is inappropriate, and you can speak to the other children's parents, to enlist their assistance in getting the teasing to stop. If your child doesn't want you to get involved, however, you probably shouldn't, because things might only get worse if you do. At school, children need much support from their teacher, school counselor, principal, and friends. Support doesn't mean getting the teacher to take punitive action toward other children; this, too, often only makes the problem worse.

Teasing may be the biggest challenge children with alopecia areata face, but it's not the only one. They have many other feelings to cope with. On the plus side, it's good to remember that children, and young children especially, can cope with more than they think. Parents worry about their child's future relationships, future career, future everything. But most children are only concerned with each day.

Children with alopecia areata want to be treated the same way they were treated before the hair loss. Parents don't need to be either more strict or more permissive. They need to treat the child as a child, perhaps adding a touch more sensitivity than before. It's a big mistake to treat the child as an unfortunate person who has a severe medical problem and is deserving of special treatment, gifts, or pity.

An important factor in determining how well a child

will adjust to alopecia areata and its treatment is how well he or she handled stress before. Again, as with adults, different children react to stress in different ways: some feel isolated and may withdraw, sleeping too much and staying away from friends and sometimes even family. Some will deny that they have the condition; that's one way of coping until they can deal with the situation differently. Others will be more accepting of their condition and prefer having it out in the open. Children can't be *forced* to react one way or the other, however, and telling them to "snap out of it" is just not helpful. Parents can explore different ways of coping with their child, and they can model good coping behavior, but if these approaches don't work and the child appears to be having real difficulty, then getting some professional counseling is an excellent idea.

When children are upset, parents and other adults can play an essential role in helping them cope. Children are aware of how adults treat them and can sense how adults feel about things. If a child sees that an adult is anxious or sad, he or she may feel anxious or sad, too. If the child sees that the adult can take the problem in stride while still doing what can be done to address the problem, that is the attitude the child is likely to adopt, too.

Some children can talk to their moms and dads about their problems, including their feelings about hair loss. But some children can't, or they can talk about all kinds of other things, but not their hair loss. Every child needs a special person to confide in, to help make sense of life experiences, whatever they are. If not a parent, this person could be a friend, a sibling, another relative, a teacher, or a counselor.

If you are the person whom the child is confiding in, listen closely. When children are asked about the positive side of having alopecia areata, they say things like: "I have a stronger personality because of it," "It helped me to grow up faster," "I don't have to get my hair cut," and "It helped me understand myself." You can be positive, too, but don't make light of the situation by listing all of the other bad possibilities in life—such as cancer—that the child has thus far avoided. And don't joke about the situation until the child indicates that he or she is ready to joke around. In addition to talking over problems, it's helpful to spend at least some of the time talking about what makes the child happy and what he or she can do well. Remind the child (but not too often) that there is always the possibility that the condition will improve.

The Family Role

Hair loss can have an effect on the child's family as well, and it's important for everyone involved to work through any emotional difficulties they may be having as a result of a child's condition. If family members are functioning well, the home will be calm and stable and the family will work well as a unit; this will help the child to cope. Family members need to put their emphasis on and give their attention to the child rather than the condition, but everyone should still learn as much as possible about the disease. The more knowledge they have about it, the more understanding and supportive they can be of the child.

Parenting a child with alopecia areata has its challenges, too. In fact, parents are often more concerned about the condition than the child. Parents often experience a whole range of emotional reactions, and most of them would exchange anything they possess in order to protect their child from what they call a hairless nightmare. Short of making the nightmare go away, there are many things that parents *can* do to deal with this condition, for themselves and for their children.

From the beginning, it is imperative that parents find a good doctor for their child, one who will tell the truth and in the truth-telling remain hopeful. Still, parents must understand that doctors are in a predicament, not in making the diagnosis of alopecia areata, but in offering any kind of prognosis. Because of the capricious nature of this disease, the hair can come and go with or without treatment. Because there is currently no cure, even if treatments work, people need to continue them, sometimes indefinitely (see chapter 3).

Although physicians can advise you on the odds of hair regrowth, it must be remembered that this is only a prediction based on what is usually seen in patients having a similar history and pattern of hair loss. Even if the odds are only one in ten that hair will regrow, hair regrowth *may* occur. Conversely, even if the odds are nine in ten that hair will regrow, it may not.

Parents often arrive at the doctor's office with inaccurate ideas about this mysterious disease. They may have noticed that their daughter's hair fell out at the same time she started menstruating, and be worried that there's some relation between the two events (none has been shown to exist). Or they may believe that their child's hair loss is caused by guilt or stress. Like adults with hair loss, the parents of children with hair loss think that if they can only find out what's *causing* it, they can reverse the condition. The best a doctor can do is kindly give you the facts about alopecia areata, present the treatment options and describe their effectiveness, remain hopeful knowing the journey can be a rough one, give you resources for coping with this condition, and refer you to a professional counselor if you or your child needs one.

After trying a variety of treatments, a doctor may tell parents that there is nothing else to do but go out and get a wig for the child. Or he or she may say something like "Go home and be grateful that your child doesn't have cancer," or (to your child) "Buy a lollipop and pretend that you're Kojak." This situation often creates some new challenges for the doctor, the parents, and the child. They don't see it coming and therefore are not prepared for it.

First, parents often feel anger at the failure of the treatments, which may translate for them into a failure on the part of the doctor. They also may be shocked by what they interpret as an authoritative dismissal. They feel unsupported and left to figure it all out themselves. They feel frustrated, helpless, hopeless, and afraid. They feel frustrated because there is no cure. They feel helpless because they can't fix it and would give anything to prevent it from getting worse. They feel hopeless because they want things to be as they used to be. And they're afraid of what's to come, fearing that the hair may never grow back.

Doctors can feel many of these same feelings, for the same reasons. And the most important person in the whole ordeal, depending on the age of the child, can feel all those same feelings, too. Alternatively, children who are not highly motivated to stick with medical treatments may be relieved that the doctor visits are coming to an end. Parents and doctors need to be sensitive to what the child wants in this situation.

Something for parents, doctors, and children to keep in mind is that everyone in the group has feelings; better still, they should talk about them out loud. Before they give up on treatment, parents need to be convinced that the doctor has done everything possible to treat the condition while at the same time being realistic about what *can* be done. If the parents think that the doctor has given up too easily, they can ask the doctor about getting a second opinion, or they can just get a second opinion on their own.

By the way, when a doctor makes comments that appear to be thoughtless or even inconsiderate of the patient's feelings, these comments are probably coming from the doctor's feeling of failure, though that doesn't excuse the behavior. You might want to calmly tell the doctor why you aren't happy with the way you and your child have been treated; if your child is old enough and you talk with the doctor honestly about your feelings in front of the child, you will be modeling good problem-solving behavior for your child that will be useful to him or her throughout life. You will also be doing the doctor a favor, since he or she may not be aware of the harmful effect those words are having. One doctor whose patient pointed out how his thoughtless comment had affected her thanked the patient sincerely and said that he would never say those words to a patient again. If you don't feel that you can talk with the doctor, you can write a brief note, which will make you feel better and, again, will help the doctor do a better job with the next patient.

As noted earlier, some parents have a harder time than their children in coping with their child's hair loss, and they may exhibit the same behaviors as someone with the disease (for example, withdrawing from friends). One reason that some parents want to avoid social situations is that other adults can sometimes be cruel in the way that children are, though mostly their "attacks" are more covert. For example, one "friend" of the mother of a young boy with alopecia areata said to her, "It must be terrible to have a child who's not perfect." The mother could say to herself "Who cares what you think?" and cross the "friend" off her holiday party list, but the comment still stung.

As important as it is to model effective coping behavior for their child, taking things in stride doesn't mean that parents have to ignore or repress their own feelings of frustration, helplessness, depression, or anger. Parents may find it helpful to talk to other parents of children with alopecia areata, to friends, or even to a professional counselor in order to learn to cope with their feelings so that they will be better able to help their child. Feelings of anxiety and guilt are not uncommon. In fact, the feeling of guilt about being responsible for your child's hair loss is common, but you can be assured that children don't blame their parents.

It's an awful thing for a parent to watch a normal, happy child suddenly change into either a quiet, withdrawn child with no confidence, or an aggressive, noisy child seeking attention. Most parents would gladly give their hair to their child if they could, and well-meaning friends might say something similar, like "I wish I could give you some of my hair, I have twice as much as I need." This approach, however, helps no one. No one feels better for the offer. What helps is listening, trying to understand, and helping the child find ways to cope.

In response to their child's emotional pain, some parents become overprotective, even keeping their child home on a windy day if she or he wears a wig. It's no wonder that parents want to protect their child, since that's the most natural instinct in the world. Still, it's better to let your child live as full a life as possible, and be there when he or she falters or falls, than to stand in the way of your child taking advantage of all that life has to offer.

Some parents say that when their child loses hair, it feels like they're losing their child. Parents who feel this way sometimes fall apart. They may try to compensate for their child's hair loss by constantly hugging the child desperately or buying (in the case of little girls) very feminine or expensive clothes. Although it is important to help children look their best, as you would with your other children, it is not a good idea to overindulge children who have the challenge of hair loss. Your energy would be better spent helping the child cope, and your money better spent as a donation for research into the disease. Don't spoil children because of their differences. It doesn't help them, it just makes them spoiled.

Brothers and sisters can also be affected by a sibling's alopecia areata. Many siblings are very close, and they may feel sad and depressed about the problems their brother or sister is having. If the children go to the same school or play with the same neighborhood playmates, the siblings may simultaneously feel embarrassed and sorry for their brother or sister. Siblings may get teased, too, about having a brother or sister with no hair. They need to be taught how to react to such teasing. Finally, sibling rivalry can rear its head under circumstances such as these, where one child in the family may be getting extra attention. Siblings may feel that they aren't as important or as well loved as the child with alopecia areata, and this can cause tension between all the children in the family. Parents need to take time for all their children. An excellent routine is to hold family meetings where everyone gets a chance to say what's on his or her mind.

Covering Up

Many children simply won't wear a wig, and they shouldn't be forced to. Wigs can be hard to adjust to, and they can be hot and sticky. Also, wigs can be pulled off by the other kids. And if the child is dead set against wearing a wig, he or she will be miserable if forced to wear one. It is important that you talk to your child about it and make the decision after discussing the pros and cons.

When little girls refuse to wear a wig, as they sometimes do, they may look like little boys, especially if they wear the same type of clothes (jeans, a T-shirt, and a cap). This can be traumatic for mothers who want to see their little girls wearing dresses, ribbons, and bows. But think: if this way of coping works for the little girl, that's good enough, and parents need to follow the child's lead in making any changes or additions in the wardrobe as time goes by and the child begins to grow up.

Children must be fitted personally for a wig (ready-made wigs won't fit). If your child is going to wear a wig, make the outing to purchase a wig a fun one. If your child is anxious about buying a wig, it may help to take the focus off that event by doing something else that day that's special, like taking in a movie with a friend. Encourage your child to play a real role in choosing a wig, and to have fun trying on all sorts of styles of "hair." Let your child pick the wig that he or she wants. A little girl may love a long, romantic wig, for example. Some children love to playact and dress up, and with wigs, they can really go to it.

The child's parent needs to provide guidance for the child about what looks good and what's affordable, and to protect the child from any thoughtless comments that adults in the wig salon might make. In fact, it's equally important to screen wig consultants for children as for adults, to weed out anyone who will make the child feel uncomfortable. Acrylic wigs are the most practical option for younger children, though some children appreciate the quality of real hair.

If your child refuses to wear a wig, don't force it. Make lots of options available, including a wig. The wig is for the child, not for anyone else. He or she may feel "weird" in anything other than a baseball cap.

On the Playground, in the Classroom

Parents who have a child with a medical condition are generally hypervigilant anyway, but it's worth saying that it's important to keep an eye on how your child is responding to having this condition. If he or she begins coming home from school upset, for example, you need to find out why. Or if your son or daughter does not want to stay after school for a special event such as an athletic meet, you will need to discuss this with him or her. It may have nothing to do with hair loss, but whatever the cause, maybe something can be done to make the situation better.

Talk about the different alternatives. Encourage your child to "brainstorm" and come up with various suggestions. Maybe he or she can help the teacher that day to keep track of the cross-country meet, or stay at school to work in the library on a story about the history of swimming in the Olympics, or interview the soccer coach for an article for the school newspaper. If your child chooses to participate in sports, you can discuss the courage it takes for people to put themselves "on the line" in a competition of any kind, and talk about the special courage it takes to swim or run with your hat off when you don't have any hair.

Perhaps this is the very situation that motivates you to educate the administration, teachers, and students in your child's class about this disease. Other children can learn about this condition and tell the bullies and teachers about it. You might consider holding a class on alopecia areata and showing the video *This Weird Thing That Makes My*

Hair Fall Out, available from NAAF. You may want to take some pamphlets along to distribute; these, too, are available from NAAF. Your child might even be able to tell the other students about alopecia areata from his or her own perspective, and you or the teacher could lead a positive discussion about the affects it has on someone's life. As noted earlier, some teachers use bald puppets to explain disabilities to classroom children, including hair loss due to cancer treatments and hair loss due to burns.

Adolescence

Adolescence can be a very difficult period in life under the best of circumstances, and hair loss makes it more so. The teenage years mark the beginning of serious peer pressures and the trying on of sex roles. Teenagers who develop alopecia areata find the condition particularly hard to deal with. They may want to change schools to escape having their friends know, or to escape teasing. An important need for them is to talk to someone they trust, and to develop social skills useful for this situation. If an adolescent is having difficulty coping with his or her hair loss—or with any other problem—then professional counseling may be helpful. Often someone who is objective and supportive and is professionally trained to help adolescents can help the teen adjust to this very upsetting condition.

Adolescents are often insecure and sensitive, and their behavior and moods can swing between the extremes of childishness and maturity. The adolescent wants to be more independent and often will assert his or her independence in front of parents. Adolescents want to be on their own, and they may feel the need to rebel against authority to get there. They don't want to be different from their friends, but hair loss makes them look and feel different.

When a young person has a medical condition it is natural for a parent to become overprotective. This can actually increase rebellion, as most adolescents object to interference from parents. Rebelling against authority is a normal part of a child's development. When it happens, be prepared to deal with it the same way you would if the child didn't have alopecia areata. Ignore it, wait until the child has calmed down, and then talk to your child. Be as tolerant and understanding as possible, and try to keep the home environment emotionally calm, stable, supportive, and loving. If the adolescent does something wrong, discuss the matter in a supportive, caring way.

Some young people with alopecia areata see it as both positive and negative—something their parents have more trouble with than they do. Shaved heads are currently a fashion statement and a symbol that makes some kids feel "cool." Many adolescents are embarrassed, however, either because they don't have normal-looking hair or because they have to wear a wig.

Making friends is very important during adolescence. Teenagers have a hard time deciding whether to tell friends, what to tell them, and which friends to tell. They may be concerned that "telling" will damage their friendships. Parents need to be aware of this so they can help. As with younger children, adolescents may welcome having teachers and parents provide a classroom lesson about alopecia areata. This can encourage a more supportive and understanding climate in the classroom and in the school.

Many misunderstood medical conditions carry a stigma, particularly during adolescence, when social relationships are most important. Adolescents with alopecia areata may wonder if anyone will ever want to date them, if they will be able to make and keep friends, if they will ever feel normal again, if they will ever get married. All teenagers wonder about these things, and having alopecia areata only makes them worry more.

Teens with alopecia areata may be reluctant to date because they are always worried that their "secret" will be found out. Or if they do tell, they are afraid that they will be rejected for not being normal. It is up to the adolescent to decide whether, when, and how to tell the date. Some feel better if they talk about it right away and not hold on to the worry. Others wait until they know the other person better.

Many adolescents with alopecia areata cope better than their parents. Parents may feel guilty and worry they could have done something to prevent their child from getting it. But for many parents, having a child with alopecia areata changes their entire outlook on life. They become more compassionate and caring and interested in learning with their son or daughter about this disease and about all kinds of other differences.

Coping

The main task with this condition is to learn how to cope with it. The psychological challenges faced by children, as with people of any age, are more important to focus on than medical treatments. In helping children to cope, the first thing to do is teach them that, other than hair loss, they are normal, healthy individuals who can do whatever is necessary to adjust to this condition. If it's necessary for them to make changes in their lifestyle, even major ones, parents can help their children to make these changes, and to believe in themselves.

The adult coping strategies described in chapter 2 can be used just as well by children. For example, support groups are a great help for kids. You can find out about any local support groups for children with alopecia areata by calling the National Alopecia Areata Foundation or your local hospital; if there isn't one, you can start one. This is very important. Children do not feel so alone with this condition when they see others who are in the same situation.

The NAAF conference has activities and sessions for children, and NAAF makes resources available to parents, as well. They will supply you with letters and articles about parents and children, brochures, pen pal lists, bimonthly newsletters, and news of support groups around the world.

With supportive parents, friends, and teachers, teenagers can live their lives like any other person of the same age. They may decide to develop expertise in an area of sports, art, music, or an academic subject. This can give a teenager a new role in the class and recognition that is not connected in any way with the amount of hair on his or her head.

It's hard work for children and teens to practice coping strategies that can help them adjust their lifestyles to fit their needs, but the rewards are worth it. We can be grateful that we are not helpless and can take action to make the most of our lives with *or without* hair.

A Day in the Life of a Person with Alopecia Areata

Mary wakes up early, feeling cold because her cap has slipped off her head again. She used to sleep with her head bare, but would wake up cold all night long. Then she tried sleeping in her wig, but she was uncomfortable and restless. Things improved after she found a soft pull-on cap, but it isn't as secure as she'd like it to be. Shivering, she pulls the cap back onto her head, pulls the covers up around her neck, and drifts off again.

At the sound of the alarm, Mary rolls out of bed. Breakfast waits while she retrieves her wig from its stand in a small cupboard by the bed and settles the familiar bulk of it on her scalp. After coffee and granola Mary dresses, then goes into the bathroom to make up her face. She used to put on her wig *after* she was dressed and made up—it seemed to be the logical way to do things—but she didn't like seeing herself in the mirror without her wig. She even had trouble concentrating on her makeup because her eyes kept being drawn to the patches of hair on her scalp.

Mary switches on the bright lights in the bathroom and pulls out the close-up mirror she uses when she applies eyelashes and eyebrows. She keeps her eyelashes and makeup in a small bag tucked away high in a cupboard. In the early days she kept them in the vanity drawer, but one day while she was having coffee with her sister and a friend, her young nephew ran into the living room brandishing her spare pack of false eyelashes and asking to play with Auntie Mary's "spiders." Mary laughs softly to herself at the memory of that day. It was a critical point for her in coping with this strange condition. Looking at little Stevie she had thought to herself, "I can't let myself be afraid of being honest with him. What have I got to lose?" So she sat Stevie down for a chat and told him she wore a wig and false eyelashes.

"Like playing pretend?" he asked, curious at the sight of her wig in her hand and her patchy head.

"Yes, just like playing pretend," she laughed. Stevie touched her wig tentatively and smiled at her.

"Let's play pretend now," he said. "You be Batman and I'll be Robin."

And that was all. What a relief. For the first time she had felt in control of her alopecia instead of victimized by it.

Mary pulls out the lashes and glue and begins the delicate task of applying them. She couldn't just glue on a strip—she found out that that looked completely unnatural—so she learned how to apply the lashes in clumps of different lengths so they looked natural. This way, too, if one section comes unstuck she'll only lose part of her "lashes," not a whole eyeful. The work is tricky, and she swears mildly as the long outer lashes go on crooked and have to be eased off and reapplied. Such fiddly things, easily damaged. "Concentrate, Mary," she tells herself. "Forget about being late for work: this is important."

Finally the lashes are in place and she can begin on her

eyebrows. These are tricky because she has some hairs on her left brow. If only they would all fall out, she could get brows tattooed on. Tattooed brows look natural except from very close up. Mary's specific dilemma is to work around her hairs to create the impression of symmetry, using only a brown pencil. And she is almost at the end of the pencil—time to stock up. Her dermatologist has suggested she have steroid shots in her eyebrow region, but fear of the pain and uncertainty about side effects have kept Mary a pencil person.

She drives to work these days. It's expensive and inconvenient to have to park all day, and she'd rather take the bus like she used to, but there were too many opportunities for wig accidents. The first wig she bought, before she discovered suction bases, had been pulled right off when someone walked by with Velcro exposed on his backpack.

At work, Mary checks her eyelashes, eyebrows, and wig in the ladies' room before going into the morning's meeting. Only her closest colleagues know her secret, and they've been sworn to secrecy. The morning passes uneventfully, except for a demanding colleague who is trying to track down the source of a shipping error. Finally he decides to talk to the data processors about the shipping program. "Sorry about all this, Mary," he says, "I'll get out of your hair now." Does that mean he knows her secret? Mary starts. Suddenly she realizes she's brooding about her hair again, while the work is piling up.

Time flies and it's ten minutes to lunch. Someone comes back into the office with dripping coat and umbrella. "What a spring we're having!" Looking out the window,

Mary sees that the streets are teeming with people carrying umbrellas. She strokes the hairless back of her neck, an unconscious nervous habit acquired when her hair first fell out. Mary has a lunch date with Michael, a man she's met recently, a friend of a friend. She hasn't dated much since her hair fell out, and she's nervous, but lunch seemed more manageable than an evening date.

She stares at the umbrellas again, watches them swaying randomly in the gusty rain. Any one of them could get caught in her wig. Surreptitiously she tugs at the side of her head. Her "hair" scarcely moves. Would it hold well enough? She had spent months trying different wigs until she found one that seemed to stay on her head as if glued. But this wig hadn't been through the umbrella test yet. Did she want to run the risk of public uncovering on the way to lunch or, worse, while walking with Michael after lunch? Finally deciding, she picks up the phone. Michael's already left, so she leaves a message apologizing for a "meeting running late."

Toward the end of day some co-workers begin arranging for a volleyball game on Friday, followed by a meal out. Mary reluctantly refuses. This isn't the first time she's backed out of social situations that might be risky for her, and she notices some of her colleagues exchanging glances. Later, her friend Trish tells Mary that people are starting to think she's a snob. "I mean, *I* know why you won't play volleyball," Trish says, "but to them you're just someone who won't loosen up and have fun with the rest of the gang." She pauses. "I could let them know about your alopecia," she volunteers.

Mary considers. "No, I can't cope with everyone knowing. I'm not ready yet. The last place I worked, people never stopped going on about it. One of the young guys kept rubbing his hair and laughing whenever I was around."

After work, Mary drops into a department store to buy that replacement eyebrow pencil—but her color isn't in stock. Only blonde or black, both of which look artificial on her. The store clerk says she can order the right shade, but it'll take two to three weeks to arrive. Mary picks again through the rows and rows of pencils. She's tried most of them and knows that they smear or wear off or lose their color. Or they're too hard, which means that instead of gliding on smoothly, they drag across her brows and make them red. She finally gives up and goes to another store, sweating in her wig, afraid to walk too fast in case she misses some dangerous cargo heading her way, like an umbrella or unaware pedestrians who might bump into her and cause some unimaginable catastrophe.

The other drugstore has also run out of her shade. Mary moves through the store, wondering what she can do about her eyebrows—until she remembers the cosmetic professional who gave a demonstration at a meeting of her support group one evening. Rosalyn had told all of them to call her any time she could be of help. Well, now is the time, Mary thinks with relief. But then she's stopped in her tracks by a tug on her head. A little boy on his father's back has his fingers stuck in her wig. Once this would have caused her panic, but these days she has learned to speak up more assertively. "Stop!" she cries, and the father apologizes and removes the boy's sticky hand. This means her wig has to be washed, and she hopes she won't have to cut sugary bits out of the style she paid so much for.

By the time she gets home the rain has ruined the set in her wig. No matter how skillfully she wields her styling comb and conditioning spray, the wig won't be at its best again until it gets its monthly reconditioning at the hair studio. She flops on the couch and switches on the television to see the screen filled with rippling, swinging hair. It's an advertisement for shampoo, of course, though it seems as if big hair plays a starring role in every single commercial and advertisement she sees these days.

Michael calls and arranges to meet her for dinner that evening. Mary starts to hum as she considers what to wear—good thing she's got a second wig!—but she's interrupted by the telephone ringing. It's her mother, calling in excitement to tell her that Mary's sister Lisa is pregnant. Mary is delighted, too, until her mother starts to sigh.

"I hope the baby will be all right," she sniffs.

"Why? Is there some problem with Lisa?"

There's silence followed by her mother's concerned statement: "I wish we knew what was wrong with *you*."

"Mom, we've been over this. It's alopecia areata, it's just hair loss. I'm not going to die from it."

"But your hair was so beautiful."

Mary puts the phone call behind her as she prepares for her date.

Dinner with Michael begins with a moment of awkwardness. The waiter pulls out the chair against the wall, and Mary has to maneuver around him deftly so she doesn't get her hair snagged on the waiter's buttons. The meal, however, is a success. Mary is pleased with herself for having the courage to date again. Getting into Michael's car, she feels a warm glow that she hasn't felt for many months. But her quiet reverie is interrupted by a clear picture of her false eyelash glue sitting by the bathroom sink. And did she leave the can of wig conditioner next to the mirror in the bathroom? She can't remember. She hopes Michael isn't the kind of man who wants to touch, especially her hair, her face, her neck, her ears. Just when she is convinced the evening will end in disaster, she is reminded that despite her anxieties, so far she has managed to handle every problem that has come her way. Her confidence returns. If this romance is meant to be, it's meant to be, and she will handle things just as well as she can.

He is moving toward her now. As much as she would like to respond to him, she ducks awkwardly around him and backs against the car door. He looks surprised. "I have to go in now; I have an early appointment in the morning."

"How about again on Friday or Saturday, then?"

"I'd love to." Once the door in her building closes behind her, she heaves a deep sigh. But it's not just that old familiar sigh of relief because nobody can see her and she can let her guard down. It goes much deeper. Something is different, something is new.

That night for the first time in many years Mary dares to dream the dreams long forgotten since the onset of her alopecia areata. If you accept the challenge and the responsibility of defining yourself, who you are and what

you can be, you will never lose. You make your own decisions, and you allow yourself to change your mind about
your decisions, if you want to. And it really doesn't matter if anyone else understands.

Sample Letters to an Insurance Company

Letter Supporting Reimbursement of the Cost of a Cranial Prosthesis for Someone with Alopecia Areata

To Whom It May Concern:

_____ has *alopecia areata,* a common disease of the hair follicle which results in loss of hair on the scalp and elsewhere. The cause of alopecia areata is unknown but is associated with an alteration in the immunological system. Patients with alopecia areata are otherwise healthy, and the condition is not contagious. It is estimated that over two million people have the disease.

Alopecia areata and its variants, alopecia totalis (loss of all scalp hair) and alopecia universalis (loss of all scalp hair and all body hair), may cause a profound alteration in the functional status of the patient. Adults have lost their jobs because of their hair loss, and they have been harassed and accused of belonging to extremist cults because of their appearance. Children have been moved from regular to special education classes and ostracized by their peers.

The disease thus represents a grave challenge to the functional status of the patient. It is not possible for the patient to lead a productive, normal life without a suitable full cranial prosthesis. The need for a full cranial prosthesis is much the same as the need for a leg prosthesis by someone with a leg amputation or the need for a breast prosthesis after a mastectomy.

It is entirely appropriate and necessary that patients with

alopecia areata, totalis, and universalis be reimbursed for their cranial prostheses.

I would be happy to provide any additional information.

Yours sincerely,

[Your doctor]

Letter Supporting Reimbursement of the Cost of Treatment for Someone with Alopecia Totalis

To Whom It May Concern:

_____has *alopecia totalis*, a severe form of a disease called alopecia areata. In alopecia totalis all hair on the entire head is lost and the skin surface becomes totally smooth and devoid of a single hair.

Alopecia areata is a common disease of the hair follicle which results in loss of hair on the scalp and body. Alopecia areata and its variants, alopecia totalis (loss of all scalp hair) and alopecia universalis (loss of all scalp hair and all body hair), may cause a profound alteration in the functional status of the patient and hence represent a grave challenge to the patient. Adults have lost their jobs because of their hair loss, and they have been harassed and accused of belonging to extremist cults because of their appearance. Children have been moved from regular to special education classes and ostracized by their peers.

The cause of alopecia areata is unknown, but it is associated with an alteration in the immunological system. Patients with alopecia areata are otherwise healthy, and the condition is not contagious. It is estimated that over two million people have alopecia areata.

Current treatment involving immunomodulating agents that stimulate hair regrowth must be continued in order to maintain the treatment's effectiveness (as is the case in many medical conditions, such as the use of antihypertensive drugs in the treatment of hypertension, or the use of insulin in diabetes mellitus). The profound and devastating effects of alopecia areata on the functional status of the patient make it necessary and reasonable that patients with the disease seek treatment.

The National Institutes of Health co-sponsored with the National Alopecia Areata Foundation a two-day Research Workshop on Alopecia Areata in 1990. This landmark workshop underscored the importance of this disease and of the need for treatments.

It is entirely appropriate and necessary that patients with alopecia areata and its variants, alopecia totalis and alopecia universalis, be reimbursed for their treatments.

I would be happy to provide any additional information.

Yours sincerely,

[Your doctor]

Letter Supporting Reimbursement of the Cost of a Cranial Prosthesis for Someone with Alopecia Universalis

To Whom It May Concern:

_____has *alopecia universalis,* the most severe form of a disease called alopecia areata. In alopecia universalis, all hair on the entire head and body is lost and the entire skin surface becomes smooth and devoid of a single hair.

Alopecia areata is a common disease of the hair follicle which results in loss of hair on the scalp and elsewhere. The cause of alopecia areata is unknown but is associated with an alteration in the immunological system. Patients with alopecia areata are otherwise healthy, and the condition is not contagious. It is estimated that over two million people have the disease.

Alopecia areata and its variants, alopecia totalis (loss of all scalp hair) and alopecia universalis (loss of all scalp hair and all body hair), may cause a profound alteration in the functional status of the patient. Adults have lost their jobs because of their hair loss, and they have been harassed and accused of belonging to extremist cults because of their appearance. Children have been moved from regular to special education classes and ostracized by their peers.

The disease thus represents a grave challenge to the functional status of the patient, and it is not possible for him or her to lead a productive, normal life without a suitable full cranial prosthesis. The need for a full cranial prosthesis is much the same as the need for a leg prosthesis by someone with a leg amputation or the need for a breast prosthesis after a mastectomy.

It is entirely appropriate and necessary that patients with alopecia areata, totalis, and universalis be reimbursed for their cranial prostheses.

I would be happy to provide any additional information.

Yours sincerely,

[Your doctor]

Resources

National Alopecia Areata Foundation (NAAF)
710 C Street, Suite 11
San Rafael, CA 94901-3853
tel. (415) 456-4644

NAAF develops public awareness of alopecia areata, raises funds for research, provides a support network and services for children and adults, and keeps patients up-to-date on new developments in research and treatment. The foundation also holds annual conferences and sends the *National Alopecia Areata Foundation Newsletter* six times annually to members of NAAF. Memberships are available beginning at $35, though the foundation adjusts the fee for those in need.

American Academy of Dermatology (AAD)
930 N. Meacham Road
Schaumburg, IL 60172-4965
tel. (708) 330-0230

AAD is a professional society of medical doctors specializing in skin diseases. The academy has a referral line, which you can call to obtain information about board-certified dermatologists near your home. (Board-certified dermatologists have been certified by the American Board of Dermatology as having passed examinations demonstrating their ability to provide competent care for people with skin diseases.) Call the AAD at the telephone number listed above and ask for "extension 505," which is the referral line. Tell the person answering the phone that you're interested in seeing a dermatologist with expertise in treating hair loss.

American Hair Loss Council (AHLC)
401 N. Michigan Avenue, 22d Floor
Chicago, IL 60611–4212
tel. (800) 274–8717

AHLC is composed of dermatologists, plastic surgeons, cosmetologists, barbers, and others who are interested in providing nonbiased information about treatment for hair loss. The council offers assistance to children as well as adults and publishes the *Hair Loss Journal* four times annually as well as a newletter. AHLC also holds an annual conference with exhibits.

A word about university medical centers. Many university medical centers—hospitals affiliated with a medical school—maintain dermatology clinics. These clinics are staffed by specialist physicians who have received additional training or who are involved in research programs designed to understand diseases and find effective treatments for them. These physicians may also be running experimental programs in which selected patients receive new treatments to test their effectiveness. The physicians in such clinics also remain up-to-date on the medical literature.

If you live near a university medical center or can visit one for a consultation, you may want to take advantage of the expertise of the physicians there. You'll want to request that your appointment be scheduled with a American Board of Dermatology–certified staff physician rather than a resident.

Some of the better-known university medical centers are Baylor University Medical Center, Dallas, Texas; the medical center of the University of California, San Francisco; the Johns

Hopkins Medical Center in Baltimore, Maryland; Massachusetts General Hospital in Boston, Massachusetts (affiliated with
the Harvard Medical School); the Medical Center of the University of Minnesota, Minneapolis; the University of Rochester
Medical Center in Rochester, New York; and the Vancouver
Hospital and Health Sciences Center, University of British Columbia, Vancouver, British Columbia. The Cleveland Clinic in
Cleveland, Ohio, and the Mayo Clinic in Rochester, Minnesota,
are excellent teaching hospitals that are not affiliated with a
medical school. There are many others, and if you live near a
big city, there's likely to be one near you.

This advice is not meant to disparage dermatologists practicing in HMOs and community hospitals, most of whom are
also highly educated professionals who keep up with advances
in research and treatment.

References

Best Overall Reviews on Alopecia Areata

Gollnick, H., et al. "Alopecia areata: pathogenesis and clinical picture." In *Hair and Hair Diseases.* Ed. C. Orfanos and R. Happle. New York: Springer, 1990.

Hordinsky, M. "Alopecia areata." In *Disorders of Hair Growth.* Ed. E. Olsen. New York: McGraw-Hill, 1994.

———, ed. *Alopecia Areata: Current Concepts.* Kalamazoo, Mich.: Upjohn Co., 1988.

Perret, C., et al. "Treatment of alopecia areata." In *Hair and Hair Diseases.* Ed. C. Orfanos and R. Happle. New York: Springer, 1990.

Price, V., et al. "Alopecia areata." *Progress in Dermatology* 25 (2): 1 (June 1991).

Rook, A., et al. "Alopecia areata." In *Diseases of the Hair and Scalp.* Cambridge, Mass.: Blackwell Scientific Publications, 1991.

Epidemiology and Course

Anderson, I. "Alopecia areata: a clinical study." *British Medical Journal* 2:1250 (1950).

Gip, L., et al. "Alopecia areata." *Acta Dermatovenereologica* 49: 180 (1969).

Ikeda, T. "A new classification of alopecia areata." *Dermatologica* 131:421 (1965).

Muller, S., et al. "Alopecia areata." *Archives of Dermatology* 88:290 (1963).

Switzer, S. "Alopecia areata in an infant." *Archives of Dermatology* 55:143 (1947).

Walker, S., et al. "Alopecia areata: a statistical study and consideration of endocrine influences." *Journal of Investigative Dermatology* 14:403 (1950).

Associated Diseases

Bergner, T., et al. "Red lunulae in severe alopecia areata." *Acta Dermatovenereologica* 72:203 (1992).

Brown, A., et al. "Ocular and testicular abnormalities in alopecia areata." *Archives of Dermatology* 118:546 (1982).

Carter, D., et al. "Alopecia areata and Down's syndrome." *Archives of Dermatology* 112:1399 (1976).

Cunliffe, W., et al. "Alopecia areata, thyroid disease and autoimmunity." *British Journal of Dermatology* 80:135 (1968).

DeWeert, J., et al. "Alopecia areata: a clinical study." *Dermatologica* 168:224 (1984).

Dhar, S., et al. "Colocalization of vitiligo and alopecia areata." *Pediatric Dermatology* 11 (1): 85 (1994).

Kanwar, A., et al. "Twenty nail dystrophy due to lichen planus in a patient with alopecia areata." *Clinical and Experimental Dermatology* 18 (3): 293 (1993).

Main, R., et al. "Smooth muscle antibodies and alopecia areata." *British Journal of Dermatology* 92:389 (1975).

McBride, A., et al. "Mosaic hair color change in alopecia areata." *Cleveland Clinic Journal of Medicine* 57:354 (1990).

Millgraum, S., et al. "Alopecia areata, endocrine function, and autoantibodies in patients 16 years and younger." *Journal of the American Academy of Dermatology* 12:57 (1987).

Muller, S., et al. "Cataracts in alopecia areata." *Archives of Dermatology* 88:290 (1963).

Orecchia, G., et al. "Lens changes in alopecia areata." *Dermatologica* 176:308 (1988).

Puavilai, S., et al. "Prevalence of thyroid diseases in patients with alopecia areata." *International Journal of Dermatology* 33 (9): 632 (1994).

Shellow, W., et al. "Profile of alopecia areata." *International Journal of Dermatology* 21:186 (1992).

Skinner, R., et al. "Alopecia areata and the presence of cytomegalovirus DNA." *JAMA* 273 (18): 1419 (1995).

Stewart, M., et al. "Alopecia universalis in an HIV positive patient: possible insight into pathogenesis." *Journal of Cutaneous Pathology* 20 (2): 180 (1993).

Taniyama, M., et al. "Simultaneous development of insulin dependent diabetes and alopecia universalis." *American Journal of Medical Science* 301:269 (1991).

Tobias, N. "Alopecia areata." *Postgraduate Medicine* 15:50 (1954).

Tosti, A., et al. "Ocular abnormalities occurring with alopecia areata." *Dermatologica* 170:69 (1985).

———. "Prevalence of nail abnormalities in children with alopecia areata." *Pediatric Dermatology* 11 (2): 112 (1994).

Wang, S. J., et al. "Increased risk for type 1 diabetes in relatives of patients with alopecia areata (AA)." *American Journal of Medical Genetics* 5193:234 (1994).

Werth, V., et al. "Incidence of alopecia areata in lupus erythematosus." *Archives of Dermatology* 128:368 (1992).

Genetics

Bereston, E., et al. "Alopecia areata in 2 brothers and 2 sisters." *Archives of Dermatology* 64:204 (1951).

Colombe, B., et al. "HLA class II alleles in longstanding alopecia totalis/alopecia universalis and longstanding patchy alopecia areata differentiate these two clinical groups." *Journal of Investigative Dermatology* 104 (5 Supp): 4S (1995).

Duvic, M., et al. "Analysis of HLA-D locus alleles in alopecia areata patients and families." *Journal of Investigative Dermatology* 104 (5 Supp): 5s (1995).

———. "HLA-D locus associations in alopecia areata." *Archives of Dermatology* 127:64 (1991).

Frentz, G., et al. "HLA DR4 in alopecia areata." *Journal of the American Academy of Dermatology* 14:129 (1986).

Friedmann, P. "Decreased autoimmunity in alopecia areata." *British Journal of Dermatology* 105:145 (1981).

Galbraith, G., et al. "Km1 allotype association with one subgroup of alopecia areata." *American Journal of Human Genetics* 44:426 (1989).

Hendren, O. "Identical alopecia areata in identical twins." *Archives of Dermatology* 60:793 (1949).

Hordinsky, M., et al. "Familial alopecia areata." *Archives of Dermatology* 120:464 (1984).

Klaber, M., et al. "Alopecia areata." *British Journal of Dermatology* 99:383 (1978).

Kuntz, B., et al. "HLA antigens in alopecia areata." *Archives of Dermatology* 113:1717 (1977).

Mikesell, J., et al. "HLA DR antigens in alopecia areata." *Cleveland Clinic Quarterly* 53:189 (1986).

Orecchia, G., et al. "HLA region involvement in the genetic predisposition to alopecia areata." *Dermatologica* 175:10 (1987).

Scerri, L., et al. "Identical twins with identical alopecia areata." *Journal of the American Academy of Dermatology* 27 (5, part 1): 766 (1992).

Selmanovitch, V., et al. "Fingerprint arches in alopecia areata." *Archives of Dermatology* 110:570 (1974).

Van der Steen, P., et al. "The genetic risk for alopecia areata in first degree relatives of severely affected patients." *Acta Dermatovenereologica* 72:373 (1992).

Zlotgorski, A., et al. "Familial alopecia areata: no linkage with HLA." *Tissue Antigens* 35:40 (1990).

Psychosomatic Aspects

Colon, E., et al. "Lifetime prevalence of psychiatric disorders in patients with alopecia areata." *Comprehensive Psychiatry* 32 (3): 245 (1991).

Greenberg, S. "Alopecia areata: a psychiatric survey." *Archives of Dermatology* 72:454 (1955).

Invernizzi, G., et al. "Life events and personality factors in patients with alopecia areata." *Medical Science Research* 15: 1219 (1987).

Koo, J., et al. "Alopecia areata and increased prevalence of psychiatric disorders." *International Journal of Dermatology* 33 (12): 849 (1994).

McAlpine, I. "Is alopecia areata psychosomatic?" *British Journal of Dermatology* 70:117 (1958).

Perini, G., et al. "Imipramine in alopecia areata: a double blind, placebo controlled study." *Psychotherapy and Psychosomatics* 61 (3/4): 195 (1994).

———. "Life events and alopecia areata." *Psychotherapy and Psychosomatics* 41:48 (1984).

Terashima, Y. "An adult case of psychogenic alopecia universalis." *Japanese Journal of Psychiatry* 43:585 (1989).

Van der Steen, P., et al. "Can alopecia areata be triggered by emotional stress?" *Acta Dermatovenereologica* 72:279 (1992).

Animal Models

Conroy, I. "Dermatopathologic signs of internal causation." *Veterinary Clinics of North America* 9 (4): 133 (1979).

Gilhar, A., et al. "The effect of topical cyclosporin on the immediate shedding of human scalp hair grafted onto nude mice." *British Journal of Dermatology* 119:767 (1988).

———. "Hair growth in scalp grafts from patients with alopecia areata and universalis grafted onto nude mice." *Archives of Dermatology* 123:44 (1987).

Oliver, R., et al. "The Debr rat model for alopecia areata." *Journal of Investigative Dermatology* 96:96 (1991).

Sundberg, J. P., et al. "Alopecia areata in aging C3H/HeJ mice." *Journal of Investigative Dermatology* 102 (6): 847 (1994).

———. "C3H/HeJ mouse model for alopecia areata." *Journal of Investigative Dermatology* 104 (5 Supp): 16s (1995).

———. "Inherited mouse mutations: models for study of alopecia." *Journal of Investigative Dermatology* 96:95s (1991).

———. *National Alopecia Areata Foundation Newsletter* (1992).

Zhang, J., et al. "Immunohistological study of the development of the cellular infiltrate in the pelage follicles of the DEBR model for alopecia areata." *British Journal of Dermatology* 130 (4): 405 (1994).

Histopathology/Immunopathology/Pathodynamics

Abdel-Naser, M., et al. "Evidence for a complement mediated inhibition and antibody dependent cellular toxicity of dermal fibroblasts in alopecia areata." *Acta Dermatovenereologica* 74 (5): 351 (1994).

Fanti, P. A., et al. "Alopecia areata: a pathological study of nonresponder patients." *American Journal of Dermatopathology* 16 (2): 167 (1994).

Gilhar, A., et al. "Response of grafts from patients with alopecia areata transplanted onto nude mice to administration of interferon gamma." *Clinical Immunology and Immunopathology* 66 (2): 120 (1993).

Goldsmith, L. "Summary of alopecia areata research workshop and future research directions." *Journal of Investigative Dermatology* 96:98s (1991).

Handjiski, B., et al. "Alkaline phosphatase activity and localization during the murine hair cycle." *British Journal of Dermatology* 131 (3): 303 (1994).

Headington, J. "The histopathology of alopecia areata." *Journal of Investigative Dermatology* 96:69s (1991).

Hoffman, R., et al. "Cytokine mRNA levels in alopecia areata before and after treatment with the contact allergen diphenylcyclopropenone." *Journal of Investigative Dermatology* 103 (4): 530 (Oct. 1994).

Hordinsky, M., et al. "Structure and function of cutaneous nerves in alopecia areata: structure and function of cutaneous nerves in alopecia areata." *Journal of Investigative Dermatology* 104 (5 Supp): 28s (1995).

———. "Suppressor cell number and function in alopecia areata." *Archives of Dermatology* 120:188 (1984).

McDonagh, A., et al. "Cytokines and dermal papilla function in alopecia areata." *Journal of Investigative Dermatology* 104 (5 Supp): 9s (1995).

———. "HLA and ICAM expression in alopecia areata in vivo and in vitro: the role of cytokines." *British Journal of Dermatology* 129 (3): 250 (1993).

Messenger, A. G., et al. "Alopecia areata: alterations in the growth cycle and correlation with follicular pathology." *British Journal of Dermatology* 114:337 (1986).

———. "Alopecia areata: light and electron microscopic pathology of the regrowing white hair." *British Journal of Dermatology* 110:155 (1984).

———. "Expression of HLA-DR by anagen hair follicles in alopecia areata." *Journal of Investigative Dermatology* 85:6 (1985).

Nickoloff, B., et al. "Aberrant ICAM-1 expression by hair follicle epithelial cells and ELAM by vascular cells are important adhesion molecule alterations in alopecia areata." *Journal of Investigative Dermatology* 96:91s (1991).

Norris, D., et al. "Immunologic cytotoxicity in alopecia areata: apoptosis of dermal papilla cells in alopecia areata." *Journal of Investigative Dermatology* 104 (5 Supp): 8s (1995).

Orecchia, G., et al. "Decreased in vitro lymphocyte stimulation and reduced sensitivity to IL-2 patients with alopecia areata." *Archives of Dermatologic Research* 280:47 (1988).

Paus, R., et al. "Is alopecia areata an autoimmune response against melanogenesis-related proteins, exposed by abnormal MHC class I expression in the anagen bulb?" *Yale Journal of Biology and Medicine* 66 (6): 541 (1993).

Randall, V., et al. "Is the dermal papilla a primary target in alopecia areata?" *Journal of Investigative Dermatology* 104 (5 Supp): 7S (1995).

Sawaya, M., et al. "CD44 expression in alopecia areata and androgenetic alopecia." *Journal of Cutaneous Pathology* 21 (3): 229 (1994).

Tobin, D., et al. "Antibodies to hair follicles in alopecia areata." *Journal of Investigative Dermatology* 102 (5): 721 (1994).

———. "Cell degeneration in alopecia areata." *American Journal of Dermatopathology* 13:248 (1991).

———. "Ultrastructural observation on the hair bulb melanocytes and melanosomes in acute alopecia areata." *Journal of Investigative Dermatology* 94:803 (1990).

Uno, H. "The histopathology of hair loss." In *Alopecia Areata: Current Concepts.* Ed. M. Hordinsky. Kalamazoo, Mich.: Upjohn Co., 1988.

Valsecchi, R., et al. "Alopecia areata and interleukin-2 receptor." *Dermatology* 184 (2): 126 (1992).

Van Baar, H., et al. "Cytokeratin expression in alopecia areata follicles." *Acta Dermatovenereologica* 74 (1): 28 (1994).

Van Scott, E. "Morphologic changes in pilosebaceous units and anagen hairs in alopecia areata." *Journal of Investigative Dermatology* 31:35 (1958).

Whiting, D. "Histopathology of alopecia areata in horizontal sections of the scalp." *Journal of Investigative Dermatology* 104 (5 Supp): 26S (1995).

Therapy

Arrazola, J., et al. "Treatment of alopecia areata with topical nitrogen mustard." *International Journal of Dermatology* 123:165 (1987).

Ashworth, J., et al. "Allergic and irritant contact dermatitis compared in the treatment of alopecia totalis and universalis: a comparison of the value of topical diphencyprone and tretinoin gel." *British Journal of Dermatology* 120:397 (1989).

Barth, J., et al. "Squaric acid dibutylester in the treatment of alopecia areata." *Dermatologica* 170:40 (1985).

Beard, H. "Social and psychological implications of alopecia areata." *Journal of the American Academy of Dermatology* 14: 696 (1986).

Bergfeld, W. Alopecia areata symposium. Ed. N. Esterly. *Paediatric Dermatology* 4:144 (1987).

Berth-Jones, J., et al. "Alopecia totalis does not respond to the vitamin D analogue calcipotriol." *Journal of Dermatologic Treatment* 1:293 (1991).

———. "Diphencyprone is not detectable in serum or urine following topical application." *Acta Dermatovenereologica* 74:312 (1994).

———. "Treatment of alopecia totalis with a combination of inosine pranobex and diphencyprone compared to each treatment alone." *Clinical and Experimental Dermatology* 16:172 (1991).

Buhl, A. "Minoxidil's action in hair follicles." *Journal of Investigative Dermatology* 96:73s (1991).

Buhl, A., et al. "Minoxidil stimulates mouse vibrissae follicles in organ culture." *Journal of Investigative Dermatology* 92: 315 (1989).

Case, P., et al. "Topical therapy of alopecia areata with squaric acid dibutylester." *Journal of the American Academy of Dermatology* 10:447 (1984).

Caserio, R. "Treatment of alopecia areata with squaric acid dibutylester." *Archives of Dermatology* 123:1037 (1987).

Claudy, A., et al. "Photochemotherapy for alopecia areata." *Acta Dermatovenereologica* (Stockholm) 60:171 (1980).

Daman, L., et al. "Treatment of alopecia areata with dinitrochlorobenzene." *Archives of Dermatology* 114:1629 (1978).

Davies, M. G., et al. "Alopecia areata arising in patients receiving cyclosporin immunosuppression." *British Journal of Dermatology* 132 (5): 835 (1995).

Deprost, Y., et al. "Dinitrochlorobenzene treatment of alopecia areata." *Archives of Dermatology* 118:542 (1982).

———. "Placebo controlled trial of topical cyclosporin in severe alopecia areata." *Lancet* 803 (Oct. 4, 1986).

———. "Treatment of severe alopecia areata by topical applications of cyclosporin: comparative trial versus placebo in 43 patients." *Transplantation Proceedings* 20 (3, Supp 4): 112 (1988).

Duhra, P., et al. "Persistent vitiligo induced by diphencyprone." *British Journal of Dermatology* 123:415 (1990).

Fanti, P., et al. "Alopecia areata: a pathologic study of nonresponder patients." *American Journal of Dermatopathology* 16 (2): 167 (1994).

Feldman, R., et al. "Absorption of some organic compounds through the skin in man." *Journal of Investigative Dermatology* 54:399 (1970).

Fiedler, V. "Alopecia areata: a review of therapy, efficacy, safety and mechanism." *Archives of Dermatology* 128:1519 (1992).

———. "Alopecia areata: current therapy." *Journal of Investigative Dermatology* 96:69s (1991).

———. "Topical minoxidil solution (1% and 5%) in the treatment of alopecia areata." *Journal of the American Academy of Dermatology* 16:737 (1987).

Fiedler-Weiss, V., et al. "Evaluation of anthralin in the treatment of alopecia areata." *Archives of Dermatology* 123:1491 (1987).

———. "Evaluation of oral minoxidil in the treatment of alopecia areata." *Archives of Dermatology* 123:1488 (1987).

———. "Topical minoxidil dose response effect in alopecia areata." *Archives of Dermatology* 122:180 (1986).

———. "Treatment resistant alopecia areata." *Archives of Dermatology* 126:756 (1990).

Flowers, F., et al. "Topical squaric acid dibutylester therapy for alopecia areata." *Cutis* 30:733 (1982).

Fransway, A., et al. "3 percent topical minoxidil compared with placebo for the treatment of chronic severe alopecia areata." *Cutis* 41:434 (1988).

Franz, T. "Percutaneous absorption of minoxidil in man." *Archives of Dermatology* 121:203 (1985).

Galbraith, G., et al. "A randomized double blind study of inosiplex therapy in patients with alopecia totalis." *Journal of the American Academy of Dermatology* 16:977 (1987).

Gebhart, W., et al. "Cyclosporin A induced hair growth in human renal allograft recipients and alopecia areata." *Archives of Dermatologic Research* 278:238 (1986).

Giannetti, A., et al. "Clinical experience on the treatment of alopecia areata with squaric acid dibutylester." *Dermatologica* 167:280 (1983).

Gilhar, A., et al. "Topical cyclosporin A in alopecia areata." *Acta Dermatovenereologica* (Stockholm) 69:252 (1989).

Gill, K., et al. "Alopecia totalis-treatment with fluocinolone acetonide." *Archives of Dermatology* 87:384 (1963).

Goldsmith, L. "Summary of alopecia areata research workshop and future research directions." *Journal of Investigative Dermatology* 96:98s (1991).

Gupta, A., et al. "Oral cyclosporin for the treatment of alopecia areata: a clinical and immunohistochemical analysis."

Journal of the American Academy of Dermatology 22:242 (1990).

Happle, R. "Antigenic competition as a therapeutic concept for alopecia areata." *Archives of Dermatologic Research* 26: 285 (1981).

———. "Topical immunotherapy in alopecia areata." *Journal of Investigative Dermatology* 96:71S (1991).

Happle, R., et al. "Contact allergy as a therapeutic tool for alopecia areata: application of squaric acid dibutylester." *Dermatologica* 7161:289 (1980).

———. "Dinitrochlorobenzene therapy for alopecia areata." *Archives of Dermatology* 114:1629 (1978).

———. "Diphencyprone in the treatment of alopecia areata." *Acta Dermatovenereologica* (Stockholm) 63:49 (1983).

Harland, C., et al. "Regression of cutaneous metastatic malignant melanoma with topical diphencyprone and oral cimetidine." *Lancet* 445 (Aug. 19, 1989).

Hatzis, J., et al. "Treatment of alopecia areata with diphencyprone." *Australasian Journal of Dermatology* 29:33 (1989).

———. "Vitiligo as a reaction to topical treatment with diphencyprone." *Dermatologica* 177:146 (1988).

Hehir, M., et al. "Alopecia areata treated with DNCB." *Clinical and Experimental Dermatology* 4:385 (1979).

Hoting, E., et al. "Therapy of alopecia areata with diphencyprone." *British Journal of Dermatology* 127:625 (1992).

Hull, S. M., et al. "Alopecia areata in children: response to treatment with diphencyprone." *British Journal of Dermatology* 125 (2): 164 (1991).

Kratka, J., et al. "Dinitrochlorobenzene: influence on the cytochrome P450 system and mutagenic effects." *Archives of Dermatologic Research* 266:315 (1979).

Lane, P., et al. "Diphencyprone." *Journal of the American Academy of Dermatology* 19:365 (1988).

Larko, O., et al. "PUVA treatment of alopecia areata." *Acta Dermatovenereologica* (Stockholm) 63:546 (1983).

Lassus, A., et al. "PUVA treatment for alopecia areata." *Dermatologica* 161:298 (1980).

Leyden, J., et al. "Treatment of alopecia areata with steroid solution." *Archives of Dermatology* 106:924 (1972).

Lowy, M., et al. "Clinical and immunologic response to isoprinosine in alopecia areata and alopecia universalis: association with autoantibodies." *Journal of the American Academy of Dermatology* 12:78 (1985).

MacDonald-Hull, S., et al. "Alopecia areata treated with diphencyprone: is allergic response necessary?" *British Journal of Dermatology* 122:716 (1990).

———. "Diphencyprone in the treatment of longstanding alopecia areata." *British Journal of Dermatology* 119:367 (1988).

———. "Post therapy relapse rate in alopecia areata after successful treatment with diphencyprone." *Journal of Dermatologic Treatment* 1:71 (1989).

———. "Successful treatment of alopecia areata using the contact allergen diphencyprone." *British Journal of Dermatology* 124:212 (1991).

Magee, K., et al. "Trial of intralesional interferon alfa in the treatment of alopecia areata." *Archives of Dermatology* 126:760 (1990).

Mitchell, A., et al. "Alopecia areata: pathogenesis and treatment." *Journal of the American Academy of Dermatology* 11:763 (1984).

———. "Topical photochemotherapy for alopecia areata." *Journal of the American Academy of Dermatology* 12:644 (1985).

Monfrecola, G., et al. "Topical hematoporphyrin plus UVA for the treatment of alopecia areata." *Photodermatology* 4:305 (1987).

Monk, B. "Induction of hair growth in alopecia totalis with diphencyprone sensitization." *Clinical and Experimental Dermatology* 14:154 (1989).

Montes, L. "Topical halcinonide in alopecia areata and alopecia totalis." *Journal of Cutaneous Pathology* 4:47 (1977).

Oken, E., et al. "Systemic steroids with or without systemic minoxidil in the treatment of alopecia areata." *Archives of Dermatology* 128:1467 (1992).

Olsen, E., et al. "Systemic steroids with or without 2% minoxidil in the treatment of alopecia areata." *Archives of Dermatology* 128 (11): 1467 (1992).

Orecchia, G., et al. "Alopecia areata and topical sensitizers: allergic response is necessary but irritation is not." *British Journal of Dermatology* 124 (5): 509 (1991).

———. "Photochemotherapy plus squaric acid dibutlylester in alopecia areata treatment." *Dermatologica* 181:167 (1990).

———. "Topical immunotherapy in children with alopecia areata." *Journal of Investigative Dermatology* 104 (5 Supp): 35S (1995).

———. "Treatment of alopecia areata with diphencyprone." *Dermatologica* 171:193 (1990).

Pascher, F., et al. "Assay of 0.2% fluocinolone acetonide cream for alopecia areata and totalis." *Dermatologica* 141:193 (1970).

Perret, C., et al. "Alopecia areata: pathogenesis and topical treatment." *International Journal of Dermatology* 29:83 (1990).

———. "Erythema multiforme-like eruptions: a rare side effect of topical immunotherapy with diphenycyclopropenone." *Dermatologica* 180:5 (1990).

———. "Treatment of alopecia areata." In *Hair and Hair Diseases*. Ed. C. Orfanos and R. Happle. New York: Springer, 1990.

Porter, D., et al. "A comparison of intra-lesional triamcinolone hexacetonide and triamcinolone acetonide in alopecia areata." *British Journal of Dermatology* 85:272 (1971).

Price, V. "Double-blind, placebo controlled evaluation of topical minoxidil in extensive alopecia areata." *Journal of the American Academy of Dermatology* 16:730 (1987).

———. "Progress in dermatology." *Bulletin of Dermatology Foundation* 25 (2): 1 (1991).

———. "Topical minoxidil in extensive alopecia areata, including 3 year followup." *Dermatologica* 175:36 (1987).

———. "Topical minoxidil (3%) in extensive alopecia areata including long term efficacy." *Journal of the American Academy of Dermatology* 16:737 (1987).

Ranchoff, R., et al. "Extensive alopecia areata: results of treatment with 3% topical minoxidil." *Cleveland Clinic Journal of Medicine* 56:149 (1989).

Roger, D., et al. "Alopecia areata occurring in a patient receiving systemic cyclosporin A." *Acta Dermatovenereologica* 74:154 (1994).

Rosenberg, E., et al. In discussion of D. Dunaway, *Alopecia Areata. Archives of Dermatology* 112:256 (1976).

Sawaya, M., et al. "Calcium-calmodulin dependent activation of glucocorticoid receptors in alopecia areata." Poster exhibit P16, American Academy of Dermatology, Dallas, Tex., 1991.

Shapiro, J. "Alopecia areata update on therapy." *Dermatologic Clinics* 11 (1): 35 (1993).

———. "Topical immunotherapy in the treatment of chronic severe alopecia areata." *Dermatologic Clinics* 11 (3): 611 (1993).

Shapiro, J., et al. "Diphencyprone and minoxidil in the treatment of alopecia areata." *Journal of the American Academy of Dermatology* 29 (5) (1993).

———. "Diphencyprone and topical minoxidil in the treatment

of chronic severe alopecia areata: a clinical and immuno-
pathologic evaluation." *Journal of Investigative Dermatology* 104 (5 Supp): 36s (1995).

Swanson, N., et al. "Topical treatment of alopecia areata: contact allergen vs. primary irritant therapy." *Archives of Dermatology* 117:384 (1981).

Thiers, B. "Isoprinosine treatment of alopecia areata." *Journal
of Investigative Dermatology* 96:72s (1991).

————. "Treatment of alopecia areata in the pediatric patient."
Alopecia areata symposium. Ed. N. Esterly. *Paediatric Dermatology* 4:136 (1987).

Tosti, A., et al. "Contact urticaria during topical immunotherapy." *Contact Dermatitis* 21:196 (1989).

————. "Therapies versus placebo in the treatment of patchy
alopecia areata." *Journal of the American Academy of Dermatology* 15:209 (1986).

————. "Thymopentin in the treatment of severe alopecia areata." *Dermatologica* 177:170 (1988).

Tritrungtasna, O., et al. "Treatment of alopecia areata with
khellin and UVA." *International Journal of Dermatology* 32
(9): 690 (1993).

Unger, W., et al. "Coritcosteroids in the treatment of alopecia
totalis." *Archives of Dermatolology* 114:1486 (1978).

Van der Steen, P., et al. "Prognostic factors in the treatment of
alopecia areata with diphenylcyclopropenone." *Journal of
the American Academy of Dermatology* 24:227 (1991).

————. "Topical immunotherapy for alopecia areata: reevalu-
ation of 139 cases after an additional follow-up period of
19 months." *Dermatology* 184 (3): 198 (1992).

————. "Treatment of alopecia areata with diphenylcyclopropenone." *Journal of the American Academy of Dermatology* 24:253 (1991).

Weisburger, E., et al. "Testing of twenty-one environmental aromatic amines or derivatives for long term toxicity or carcinogenicity." *Journal of Environmental Pathology and Toxicology* 2:325 (1978).

Weiss, V., et al. "Alopecia areata treated with topical minoxidil." *Archives of Dermatology* 120:457 (1984).

Whiting, D. "The treatment of alopecia areata." *Cutis* 40:248 (1987).

Wilkerson, M., et al. "Assessment of diphenylcyclopropenone for photochemical induced mutagenicity in the Ames assay." *Journal of the American Academy of Dermatology* 17:606 (1987).

———. "Contaminants of dinitrochlorobenzene." *Journal of the American Academy of Dermatology* 9:554 (1983).

———. "Diphenylcyclopropenone: examination for potential contaminants, mechanism of sensitization and photochemical stability." *Journal of the American Academy of Dermatology* 11:802 (1984).

Winter, R., et al. "Prednisone therapy for alopecia areata." *Archives of Dermatology* 112:1549 (1976).

Yuan-Pei Shi. "Topical minoxidil in the treatment of alopecia areata and male pattern alopecia." *Archives of Dermatology* 122:506 (1986).

Index

adolescents with alopecia areata, 137–39

affirmations, 19

alopecia areata: acute phase, 56; in adolescents, 137–39; advice for people with, 78; and alternative medicine, 80–82; ancient remedies, 78–79; androgenic, 47; anxiety associated with, 4–5, 41–42; attitude toward, 28–30; as autoimmune disease, 48–52; causes of, 47–52; chronic, 56–57; conditions accompanying, 52–54; and cytomegalovirus, 52; day in the life of a person with, 142–49; diagnosis of, 16, 56–58; educating others about, 35–36; emotional reactions to, 19–20; fears associated with, 32–33; genetic factors, 48, 51–52, 54–55; impact on family and friends, 17; as life-changing event, 18–22; loss and grieving associated with, 8–10; medical treatment for, 25–28; miracle cures, 78–79; of the nails, 45; origin of name, 1; patterns of, 57; prognosis, 58–61; psychological impact of, 2–8, 15, 17–18; remission of, 60; research on, 51–52; and sexuality, 38–42; stress associated with, 30–32; subacute phase, 56; and thyroid disease, 53; treatment for, 61–77, 82–83; and trichoquackery, 79–80; unpredictability of, 1–2; videotape on, 26, 136–37. *See also* children with alopecia areata; treatments

alopecia-masking lotion, 90

alopecia totalis, 2, 44

alopecia universalis, 2, 44–45

American Academy of Dermatology, 155–56

American Academy of Dermatology White Paper on Alopecia Areata, 105, 108

American Hair Loss Council, 156

anagen phase, 46

androgenic alopecia, 47, 88

anthralin cream, 68, 76

anxiety, associated with alopecia areata, 4–5, 41–42

atopy, 53

attitude, adjusting, 28–30

autoimmune disease, alopecia areata as, 48–52

betamethasone dipropionate, 67, 76

biopsy of scalp, 58

bullying, 123–24

catagen phase, 46

children with alopecia areata, 120–21; adolescents, 137–39; educating of, 123; and educating other children about alopecia,

LIBRARY OF CONGRESS CATALOGING-IN-PUBLICATION DATA

Thompson, Wendy J. A.
    Alopecia areata : understanding and coping with hair loss / Wendy
Thompson and Jerry Shapiro; foreword by Vera H. Price.
        p.   cm.
    Includes bibliographical references and index.
    ISBN 0-8018-5352-4 (hc : alk. paper)
        1. Alopecia areata.   I. Shapiro, Jerry.   II. Title.
RL155.5.T47   1996
616.5'46—dc20   96-33971